Airway Management

Editors

LYNETTE MARK
MAREK A. MIRSKI
PAUL W. FLINT

ANESTHESIOLOGY CLINICS

www.anesthesiology.theclinics.com

Consulting Editor
LEE A. FLEISHER

JUNE 2015 • Volume 33 • Number 2

ELSEVIER

1600 John F. Kennedy Boulevard • Suite 1800 • Philadelphia, Pennsylvania, 19103-2899

http://www.theclinics.com

ANESTHESIOLOGY CLINICS Volume 33, Number 2
June 2015 ISSN 1932-2275, ISBN-13: 978-0-323-38876-4

Editor: Jennifer Flynn-Briggs
Developmental Editor: Susan Showalter

Anesthesiology Clinics (ISSN 1932-2275) is published quarterly by Elsevier Inc., 360 Park Avenue South, New York, NY 10010-1710. Months of issue are March, June, September, and December. Periodicals postage paid at New York, NY and at additional mailing offices. Subscription prices are $160.00 per year (US student/resident), $330.00 per year (US individuals), $400.00 per year (Canadian individuals), $533.00 per year (US institutions), $674.00 per year (Canadian institutions), $225.00 per year (Canadian and foreign student/resident), $455.00 per year (foreign individuals), and $674.00 per year (foreign institutions). To receive student and resident rate, orders must be accompanied by name of affiliated institution, date of term, and the *signature* of program/residency coordinator on institutions letterhead. Orders will be billed at individual rate until proof of status is received. Foreign air speed delivery is included in all *Clinics'* subscription prices. All prices are subject to change without notice. POSTMASTER: Send address changes to *Anesthesiology Clinics,* Elsevier Health Sciences Division, Subscription Customer Service, 3251 Riverport Lane, Maryland Heights, MO 63043. Customer Service (orders, claims, online, change of address): Elsevier Health Sciences Division, Subscription Customer Service, 3251 Riverport Lane, Maryland Heights, MO 63043. **Tel:1-800-654-2452 (U.S. and Canada); 314-447-8871 (outside U.S. and Canada). Fax: 314-447-8029. E-mail: journalscustomerservice-usa@elsevier.com (for print support); journalsonlinesupport-usa@elsevier.com (for online support).**

Reprints. For copies of 100 or more of articles in this publication, please contact the Commercial Reprints Department, Elsevier Inc., 360 Park Avenue South, New York, NY 10010-1710. Tel.: 212-633-3874; Fax: 212-633-3820; E-mail: reprints@elsevier.com.

Anesthesiology Clinics, is also published in Spanish by McGraw-Hill Inter-americana Editores S. A., P.O. Box 5-237, 06500 Mexico D. F., Mexico.

Anesthesiology Clinics, is covered in *MEDLINE/PubMed (Index Medicus), Current Contents/Clinical Medicine, Excerpta Medica, ISI/BIOMED,* and *Chemical Abstracts.*

Contributors

CONSULTING EDITOR

LEE A. FLEISHER, MD, FACC, FAHA
Robert D. Dripps Professor and Chair of Anesthesiology and Critical Care, Professor of Medicine, Perelman School of Medicine, University of Pennsylvania School of Medicine, Philadelphia, Pennsylvania

EDITORS

LYNETTE MARK, MD
Associate Professor, Departments of Anesthesiology and Critical Care Medicine, and Otolaryngology–Head and Neck Surgery; Director, Difficult Airway Response Team (DART) Program, The Johns Hopkins University School of Medicine, Baltimore, Maryland

MAREK A. MIRSKI, MD, PhD
Department of Anesthesiology and Critical Care Medicine, Neurology, Neurosurgery, Johns Hopkins University School of Medicine, Baltimore, Maryland

PAUL W. FLINT, MD, FACS
Otolaryngology–Head and Neck Surgery, Oregon Health and Science University, Portland, Oregon

AUTHORS

JASON A. AKULIAN, MD, MPH
Director, Section of Interventional Pulmonology, Assistant Professor of Medicine, Division of Pulmonary and Critical Care Medicine, University of North Carolina at Chapel Hill, Chapel Hill, North Carloina

CARLOS A. ARTIME, MD
Assistant Professor, Department of Anesthesiology, University of Texas Medical School at Houston, Houston, Texas

PAUL BAKER, MBChB, MD, FANZCA
Clinical Senior Lecturer, Department of Anaesthesiology, The University of Auckland, Auckland, New Zealand

MONIKA CHMIELEWSKA, DO
Instructor, Department of Otolaryngology–Head and Neck Surgery, Johns Hopkins Hospital, Baltimore, Maryland

RICHARD M. COOPER, MSc, MD, FRPCP
Professor, Department of Anesthesia, University of Toronto; Department of Anesthesia and Pain Management, Toronto General Hospital, Toronto, Ontario, Canada

D. JOHN DOYLE, MD, PhD
Professor of Anesthesiology, Case Western Reserve University Staff Anesthesiologist, Department of General Anesthesiology, Cleveland Clinic Foundation; Chief, Department of General Anesthesiology, Anesthesiology Institute, Cleveland Clinic Abu Dhabi, Abu Dhabi, United Arab Emirates

JESSICA FEINLEIB, MD, PhD
Staff Anesthesiologist, West Haven VA, West Haven; Assistant Professor of Anesthesiology, Yale University School of Medicine, New Haven, Connecticut

DAVID FELLER-KOPMAN, MD
Director, Bronchoscopy and Interventional Pulmonology, Section of Interventional Pulmonology, Division of Pulmonary and Critical Care, Associate Professor of Medicine, Otolaryngology–Head and Neck Surgery, Johns Hopkins Hospital, Johns Hopkins University, Baltimore, Maryland

LORRAINE FOLEY, MD, MBA
Winchester Anesthesia Associates, Winchester Hospital; Clinical Assistant Professor of Anesthesia, Tufts School of Medicine, Boston, Massachusetts

CARIN A. HAGBERG, MD
Joseph C. Gabel Professor and Chair, Department of Anesthesiology, University of Texas Medical School at Houston, Houston, Texas

ALEXANDER T. HILLEL, MD
Assistant Professor, Department of Otolaryngology–Head and Neck Surgery, Johns Hopkins Hospital, Baltimore, Maryland

DAWN M. LARSON, MD
Department of Anesthesiology and Perioperative Medicine, Oregon Health and Science University, Portland, Oregon

GARY LINKOV, MD
Senior Resident, Temple University Hospital, Philadelphia, Pennsylvania

LYNETTE MARK, MD
Associate Professor, Departments of Anesthesiology and Critical Care Medicine, and Otolaryngology–Head and Neck Surgery; Director, Difficult Airway Response Team (DART) Program, The Johns Hopkins University School of Medicine, Baltimore, Maryland

ROSS P. MARTINI, MD
Department of Anesthesiology and Perioperative Medicine, Oregon Health and Science University, Portland, Oregon

RYAN K. MEACHAM, MD
Fellow, Department of Otolaryngology, Oregon Health Sciences University, Portland, Oregon

KARLA O'DELL, MD
Assistant Professor, Laryngology, Voice, Airway and Swallowing Disorders, Department of Otolaryngology, Head and Neck Surgery, Keck School of Medicine, University of Southern California, Los Angeles, California

VINCIYA PANDIAN, PhD
Assistant Professor, Department of Anesthesiology and Critical Care Medicine, Johns Hopkins Hospital, Baltimore, Maryland

JOSHUA SCHINDLER, MD
Associate Professor, Department of Otolaryngology, Oregon Health Sciences University, Portland, Oregon

AHMED M.S. SOLIMAN, MD
Professor and Associate Chairperson, Department of Otolaryngology–Head and Neck Surgery; Director, Voice, Airway & Swallowing Center, Temple University School of Medicine, Philadelphia, Pennsylvania

TRACEY L. STIERER, MD
Assistant Professor, Anesthesiology and Critical Care Medicine; Otolaryngology, Head and Neck Surgery, Johns Hopkins Medicine, Baltimore, Maryland

BRADFORD D. WINTERS, PhD, MD
Assistant Professor, Department of Anesthesiology and Critical Care Medicine, Johns Hopkins Hospital, Baltimore, Maryland

LONNY YARMUS, DO
Program Director, Section of Interventional Pulmonology, Assistant Professor of Medicine, Division of Pulmonary and Critical Care, Johns Hopkins Hospital, Johns Hopkins University, Baltimore, Maryland

JOSHUA SCHINDLER, MD
Associate Professor, Department of Otolaryngology, Oregon Health Sciences University, Portland, Oregon

AHMED M.S. SOLIMAN, MD
Professor and Associate Chairperson, Department of Otolaryngology–Head and Neck Surgery; Director, Voice, Airway & Swallowing Center, Temple University School of Medicine, Philadelphia, Pennsylvania

TRACEY L. STIERER, MD
Assistant Professor of Anesthesiology and Critical Care Medicine, Otolaryngology, Head and Neck Surgery, Johns Hopkins Medicine, Baltimore, Maryland

BRADFORD D. WINTERS, PhD, MD
Assistant Professor, Department of Anesthesiology and Critical Care Medicine, Johns Hopkins Hospital, Baltimore, Maryland

LONNY YARMUS, DO
Program Director, Section of Interventional Pulmonology; Assistant Professor of Medicine, Division of Pulmonary and Critical Care, Johns Hopkins Hospital, Johns Hopkins University, Baltimore, Maryland

Contents

ANESTHESIOLOGY CLINICS

THE CLINICS ARE AVAILABLE ONLINE!
Access your subscription at:
www.theclinics.com

ANESTHESIOLOGY CLINICS

FORTHCOMING ISSUES

September 2015
Geriatric Anesthesia
Mark D. Neuman and Charles Brown,
Editors

December 2015
Value-Based Care
Lee A. Fleisher, Editor

March 2016
Preoperative Evaluation
Debra Pulley and
Deborah C. Richman, Editors

RECENT ISSUES

March 2015
Anesthetic Care for Abdominal Surgery
Timothy Miller and Michael Scott, Editors

December 2014
Orthopedic Anesthesiology
Nabil M. Elkassabany and
Edward R. Mariano, Editors

September 2014
Vascular Anesthesia
Charles Hill, Editor

June 2014
Ambulatory Anesthesiology
Jeffrey L. Apfelbaum
and Thomas W. Cutter, Editors

RELATED INTEREST

Surgical Clinics April 2015 (Vol. 95, Issue 2)
Clinics in Chest Medicine March 2015 (Vol.36, Issue 1)
Primary Care: Clinics in Office Practice, March 2015 (Vol. 42, Issue 1)
Critical Care Clinics April 2015 (Vol. 31, Issue 2)

Foreword
Airway Management

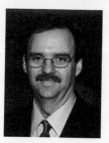

Lee A. Fleisher, MD, FACC, FAHA
Consulting Editor

As anesthesiologists, management of the airway is a critical component of our daily activities. Our ability to evaluate and better manage the airway has evolved tremendously since the Closed Claims Analysis identified some of the key factors that were associated with complications and failed intubations. In this issue of *Anesthesiology Clinics*, both the evaluation and the new management techniques are explored. Guidelines, educational issues, and communication are also highlighted. Among the unique challenges is the management of the airway in the professional voice patient, outlined by one of the editors. Therefore, this issue provides up-to-date information on one of the primary activities.

In choosing a group of guest editors for this issue, I am pleased to have a multidisciplinary group in Drs Lynette Mark, Marek Mirski, and Paul Flint. Lynette Mark, MD is an Associate Professor of Anesthesiology and Critical Care Medicine and Otolaryngology–Head and Neck Surgery at the Johns Hopkins Medical Institutions. She founded and chaired the Anesthesia Advisory Council to the nonprofit MedicAlert Foundation and in 1992 created the National Difficult Airway/Intubation Registry. Dr Mark was also a founding member of the Society for Airway Management (SAM). Marek Mirski, MD, PhD is the Thomas and Dorothy Toung Professor of Anesthesiology and Critical Care Medicine and is also Professor of Neurology and Neurosurgery at Johns Hopkins Medical Institution. He was for many years the Director of Johns Hopkins Neuroscience Critical Care Division, Chief of Neuroanesthesiology, and Director of the Anesthesiology Clinical Research Program. Paul Flint, MD is Professor and Chair of Otolaryngology–Head and Neck Surgery at Oregon Health and Science

Anesthesiology Clin 33 (2015) xiii–xiv
http://dx.doi.org/10.1016/j.anclin.2015.03.002
1932-2275/15/$ – see front matter © 2015 Published by Elsevier Inc.

anesthesiology.theclinics.com

University. He is also a founding member of SAM and a Senior Editor of the *Textbook of Otolaryngology–Head and Neck Surgery*. Together, they have brought us a comprehensive issue of *Anesthesiology Clinics* on an important topic.

Lee A. Fleisher, MD, FACC, FAHA
Anesthesiology and Critical Care
Perelman School of Medicine
University of Pennsylvania
Philadelphia, PA 19104, USA

E-mail address:
Lee.fleisher@uphs.upenn.edu

Preface

Airway Management

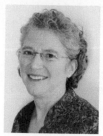
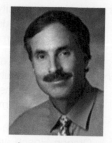
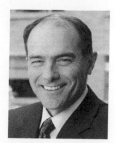

Lynette Mark, MD   Marek A. Mirski, MD, PhD   Paul W. Flint, MD, FACS

Editors

Any single life lost in airway management is one life too many.
—Andranik (Andy) Ovassapian (2009)

"Airway Management" is dedicated to Dr Andranik (Andy) Ovassapian: a mentor, friend, and colleague to generations of clinicians during the nearly half century that he practiced anesthesiology. Andy is probably best credited with establishing fiber-optic intubation techniques as "gold standards" for difficult airway management, assisting in the development of the American Society of Anesthesiologists Practice Guidelines for Management of the Difficult Airway, helping create the MedicAlert National Airway/Intubation Registry, founding the Society for Airway Management or SAM, supporting other countries in their efforts to create airway management societies, and most importantly, fostering cross-fertilization of all disciplines engaged in airway management. Andy was to be a co-guest editor in a 2009 *Anesthesiology Clinics* Airway Management issue, but with his untimely death in 2010, the issue was suspended. Many of the topics presented here are ones that Andy identified as significant for both the novice and the expert to master in efforts to *"prevent airway deaths— even if it is just one death."*

In our experience, airway management approached as a team effort provides the safest environment for our patients. This has been demonstrated through the development of the Difficult Airway Response Team or DART Program presented in this issue. Adapting this approach insures that equipment, personnel, and information are aligned and available for managing the known and unknown difficult airway. Airway Management presents a multidisciplinary approach to clinical issues that have been reviewed and updated to reflect the current state of clinical practices. This issue is organized into 4 broad areas: (1) practice guidelines, assessment, and preparation; (2) specialty considerations; (3) emergency airway response teams, expertise, and competency; and (4) communications about airway management and national and international airway registries.

Anesthesiology Clin 33 (2015) xv–xvi
http://dx.doi.org/10.1016/j.anclin.2015.03.001
1932-2275/15/$ – see front matter © 2015 Published by Elsevier Inc.

anesthesiology.theclinics.com

We hope that practitioners will read these articles—written by a group of multidisciplinary international experts—and adapt clinical pearls and wisdom into everyday airway management practice.

Lynette Mark, MD
Johns Hopkins University School of Medicine
1800 Orleans Street, ZB 6214
Baltimore, MD 21287, USA

Marek A. Mirski, MD, PhD
Johns Hopkins University School of Medicine
1800 Orleans Street, Phipps 455B
Baltimore, MD 21287, USA

Paul W. Flint, MD, FACS
Oregon Health and Science University
3181 SW Sam Jackson Park Road, PV01
Portland, OR 97239-3098, USA

E-mail addresses:
lmark@jhmi.edu (L. Mark)
mmirski1@jhmi.edu (M.A. Mirski)
flint@ohsu.edu (P.W. Flint)

Is There a Gold Standard for Management of the Difficult Airway?

Carlos A. Artime, MD, Carin A. Hagberg, MD*

KEYWORDS

- Airway management • Algorithms • Difficult airway • Intubation • Practice guidelines

KEY POINTS

- The American Society of Anesthesiologists' (ASA) PRACTICE GUIDELINES FOR THE MANAGEMENT OF THE DIFFICULT AIRWAY are systematically developed using a comprehensive evaluation of the medical literature, opinion surveys, and critical review by expert consultants and opinion surveys from the ASA community at large.
- Several different national anesthesia societies (including the United Kingdom, Canada, France, Germany, and Italy) have published their own guidelines for managing the difficult airway that are based on literature reviews and expert opinion.
- No other specialties involved in airway management have produced their own guidelines for difficult airway management based on a systematic review of the literature.
- No evidence exists to support one set of guidelines over another as a gold standard.

INTRODUCTION

For the clinician involved in airway management, the difficult airway remains one of the most relevant and challenging clinical circumstances owing to the potentially grave implications of failing to establish a patent airway. Therefore, numerous practice guidelines have been developed to assist clinicians in managing the difficult airway; several algorithms have been devised to assimilate these guidelines into stepwise decision trees that a practitioner can use when faced with this clinical situation.

The concept of a gold standard in medicine dates back to 1979 and has since been used innumerable times in the literature.[1] Although a gold standard has been defined by some as an ultimate standard that is beyond reproach,[2] it is more commonly used to

Much of the content in this article has been reprinted from Berkow L, Sakles J (editors). Cases in emergency airway management. Cambridge, UK: Cambridge University Press, 2015 (in press). Copyright © 2015 Cambridge University Press.
Department of Anesthesiology, University of Texas Medical School at Houston, 6431 Fannin Street, MSB 5.020, Houston, TX 77030, USA
* Corresponding author.
E-mail address: carin.a.hagberg@uth.tmc.edu

Anesthesiology Clin 33 (2015) 233–240
http://dx.doi.org/10.1016/j.anclin.2015.02.011
anesthesiology.theclinics.com

describe the best available practice.[3] *Standards of care* refer to a minimum standard that can be expected from a medical practitioner in a given clinical situation. Most clinical gold standards are determined by large randomized controlled trials, systematic reviews, and meta-analyses. The nature of difficult airway management, however, does not provide a practical way of comparing different guidelines or algorithms. This article reviews several different guidelines and algorithms and the evidence supporting them.

THE AMERICAN SOCIETY OF ANESTHESIOLOGISTS' PRACTICE GUIDELINES FOR MANAGEMENT OF THE DIFFICULT AIRWAY

In 1990, the American Society of Anesthesiologists (ASA) formed the Task Force on Management of the Difficult Airway in response to an analysis of the ASA's Closed Claims database that showed that adverse respiratory events were responsible for a plurality of settled or awarded claims related to unfavorable anesthetic outcomes and that death or hypoxic brain damage occurred in most such cases.[4]

The product of that task force was the ASA's 1993 "Practice Guidelines for Management of the Difficult Airway," which sought to "facilitate the management of the difficult airway and reduce the likelihood of adverse outcomes."[5] These guidelines delineated recommendations for evaluation of the airway, basic preparation for difficult airway management, and a strategy for intubating the difficult airway centered on a difficult airway algorithm (DAA). The practice guidelines have since undergone 2 revisions: first in 2003, which, among other changes, incorporated the use of the laryngeal mask airway (LMA) into the algorithm, and most recently in 2013.[6] Among the most recent modifications are the replacement of LMA with supraglottic airway (SGA) to reflect the growing number of SGAs available in clinical practice and the addition of video-assisted laryngoscopy (VAL) as both an initial approach to intubation (awake or following induction of general anesthesia) and after failed intubation when face mask or SGA ventilation is adequate.

The ASA's practice guidelines are systematically developed using a comprehensive evaluation of the medical literature, opinion surveys and critical review by expert consultants, and opinion surveys from the ASA community at large. Evidence from original studies published in peer-reviewed journals was aggregated and systematically reported by the strength and quality of the research design and study findings.

A prominent focus of the ASA's practice guidelines is the formation of organized, preplanned strategies for airway management, including a preemptive evaluation of the airway intended to detect a potentially difficult airway ahead of time. Advanced recognition enables the practitioner to formulate a specific management plan for patients and provides an opportunity to secure the airway before induction of general anesthesia (ie, awake intubation). The likelihood of difficulty with one or more of the following should be assessed: patient cooperation or consent, mask ventilation, SGA placement, laryngoscopy, intubation, and surgical airway access.

The ASA's DAA (**Fig. 1**) is the practice guidelines' recommended strategy for intubation of the difficult airway. It begins with a consideration of the relative clinical merits and feasibility of 4 basic management choices: (1) awake intubation versus intubation after induction of general anesthesia, (2) noninvasive versus invasive techniques (ie, surgical or percutaneous airway) for the initial approach to intubation, (3) VAL as an initial approach to intubation, and (4) preservation versus ablation of spontaneous ventilation.

The ASA's DAA can seem confusing at first glance because it does not follow a linear decision-making tree, as the advanced cardiovascular life support algorithms do. However, it can be better understood and remembered by considering it as 3 separate scenarios: (1) predicted difficult airway (awake intubation), (2) difficult intubation

DIFFICULT AIRWAY ALGORITHM

1. **Assess the likelihood and clinical impact of basic management problems:**
   - Difficulty with patient cooperation or consent
   - Difficult mask ventilation
   - Difficult supraglottic airway placement
   - Difficult laryngoscopy
   - Difficult intubation
   - Difficult surgical airway access

2. **Actively pursue opportunities to deliver supplemental oxygen throughout the process of difficult airway management.**

3. **Consider the relative merits and feasibility of basic management choices:**
   - Awake intubation *vs.* intubation after induction of general anesthesia
   - Non-invasive technique *vs.* invasive techniques for the initial approach to intubation
   - Video-assisted laryngoscopy as an initial approach to intubation
   - Preservation *vs.* ablation of spontaneous ventilation

4. **Develop primary and alternative strategies:**

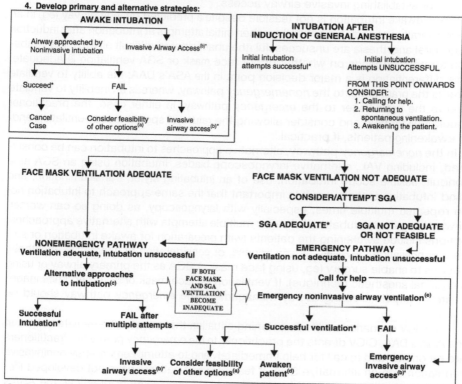

*Confirm ventilation, tracheal intubation, or SGA placement with exhaled CO$_2$.

a. Other options include (but are not limited to): surgery utilizing face mask or supraglottic airway (SGA) anesthesia (e.g., LMA, ILMA, laryngeal tube), local anesthesia infiltration or regional nerve blockade. Pursuit of these options usually implies that mask ventilation will not be problematic. Therefore, these options may be of limited value if this step in the algorithm has been reached via the Emergency Pathway.

b. Invasive airway access includes surgical or percutaneous airway, jet ventilation, and retrograde intubation.

c. Alternative difficult intubation approaches include (but are not limited to): video-assisted laryngoscopy, alternative laryngoscope blades, SGA (e.g., LMA or ILMA) as an intubation conduit (with or without fiberoptic guidance), fiberoptic intubation, intubating stylet or tube changer, light wand, and blind oral or nasal intubation.

d. Consider re-preparation of the patient for awake intubation or canceling surgery.

e. Emergency non-invasive airway ventilation consists of a SGA.

Fig. 1. The ASA's DAA. (*From* Apfelbaum JL, Hagberg CA, Caplan RA, et al. Practice guidelines for management of the difficult airway: an updated report by the American Society of Anesthesiologists Task Force on Management of the Difficult Airway. Anesthesiology 2013;118:257; with permission.)

with adequate ventilation, and (3) difficult intubation without adequate ventilation (the *cannot intubate, cannot ventilate* [CICV] scenario).

In the predicted difficult airway, awake intubation is generally indicated for the following reasons: (1) patency of the airway is maintained through upper pharyngeal muscle tone; (2) spontaneous ventilation is maintained; and (3) awake patients are easier to intubate because the larynx moves to a more anterior position after induction of anesthesia. Awake intubation may be attempted through noninvasive or invasive methods (eg, surgical airway, percutaneous airway, or retrograde intubation). In the ASA's DAA, several options are suggested if awake intubation fails, including canceling and postponing surgery, performing surgery using a face mask or SGA ventilation (if these are not predicted to be difficult), using a regional anesthetic technique, or establishing invasive airway access.

When awake intubation is not feasible despite a predicted difficult airway (eg, in an uncooperative or pediatric patient) or when initial attempts at intubation after induction of general anesthesia are unsuccessful (the unanticipated difficult airway), the intubation strategy depends on whether or not face mask or SGA ventilation is adequate. This differentiation is a major decision point in the ASA's DAA; the ability to ventilate directs the practitioner to the *nonemergency* pathway, whereas an inability to ventilate directs the practitioner to the *emergency* pathway. In either case, the practitioner should call for help and consider allowing the return of spontaneous ventilation and/or awakening patients, if practical.

In the *nonemergency* pathway, alternative approaches to intubation can be considered, including VAL, alternative laryngoscope blades, intubation using an SGA as a conduit, flexible scope intubation, use of an intubating stylet, transillumination, and blind intubation techniques. It is important that the same approach to intubation not be repeated multiple times, especially with laryngoscopy, as doing so can worsen airway integrity. If intubation fails after multiple attempts with alternative approaches, options include awakening the patients (with preparation for awake intubation or surgery cancellation), invasive airway access, or consideration of alternative anesthetic options to enable surgery (eg, using face mask or SGA as the primary airway or using a regional anesthetic technique). If ventilation via face mask or SGA becomes inadequate at any time during airway management, the *emergency* pathway should be followed.

The CICV scenario is a life-threatening situation that requires immediate action. In the ASA's DAA, CICV directs the practitioner to the *emergency* pathway. Practitioners are recommended to call for help immediately and to attempt emergency noninvasive ventilation with an alternative SGA, if feasible (ie, if patients have not developed life-threatening hypoxemia). If SGA placement is not successful or practical, the ASA's DAA recommends obtaining emergency invasive airway access (ie, surgical or percutaneous airway or transtracheal jet ventilation).

The ASA's practice guidelines and the ASA's DAA have been subject to criticism for various reasons, particularly for the difficulty practitioners have following the multiple decision points. The broad, comprehensive nature of the recommended techniques at various points in the algorithm has also been critiqued as being insufficiently specific to be of use in a true airway emergency. These guidelines, however, are intended to be basic recommendations and not standards of care or absolute requirements.[7] Rather, the recommendations found in the ASA's practice guidelines should be used to help formulate a plan for airway management and should be adapted to reflect the specific skillset of the practitioner as well as individual patient factors.

The ASA's DAA has also been criticized for beginning with a failure to intubate, in effect assuming that the primary intention of the airway practitioner is to intubate the trachea.[8] Considering that difficulty with face mask ventilation or SGA placement is often the initial difficulty encountered, the algorithm may then direct the practitioner toward interventions that have already proven ineffective. Other criticisms include a lack of recommendations for the assessment of aspiration risk and the use of muscle relaxation as well as various other minor inconsistencies, such as the inclusion of retrograde intubation as an option for emergency invasive airway access in the *emergency* pathway.[9]

OTHER NATIONAL ANESTHESIA SOCIETY GUIDELINES

In addition to the ASA, several different national anesthesia societies have published their own guidelines for the management of the difficult airway, including the Difficult Airway Society (DAS) from the United Kingdom, the Canadian Airway Focus Group (CAFG), the French Society of Anesthesia and Intensive Care (SFAR), the German Society of Anesthesiology and Intensive Care Medicine (DGAI), and the Italian Society for Anesthesia and Intensive Care (SIAARTI).[10–14]

Like the ASA's guidelines, the CAFG and SIAARTI guidelines' methodologies include a systematic review of the literature with classification of level of evidence. The guidelines published by the DAS, SFAR, and DGAI include literature reviews but do not aggregate and classify evidence in a systematic fashion.

With the exception of the DAS' guidelines, all of these guidelines include recommendations for the prediction of the difficult airway and suggest awake intubation as a management strategy. All of the practice guidelines include algorithms for both unanticipated difficult intubation with adequate oxygenation and the CICV scenario. Commonalities include a focus on awakening patients if intubation is difficult but ventilation is adequate, using an SGA as a rescue for difficult mask ventilation, and performing an emergency surgical airway in the CICV scenario. The primary differences in these algorithms are in specific details, such as the number of intubation attempts suggested, the specific alternate devices recommended for difficult intubation, and the organization of the algorithm. Like the ASA's algorithm, the Italian, French, and German guidelines incorporate all scenarios into one algorithm, whereas the guidelines from the DAS and CAFG have distinct algorithms for specific scenarios.

INSTITUTIONAL ALGORITHMS

A limitation of the guidelines and algorithms presented thus far is a lack of validation in clinical trials. Although a recent analysis of the ASA's Closed Claims database showed that the incidence of adverse respiratory events at induction has decreased since the introduction of the ASA's DAA,[15] it is difficult to assign sole benefit to the adoption of the ASA practice guidelines' recommendations.

Various institutional algorithms have been devised and many have been evaluated in clinical trials. These institutional algorithms differ from national society guidelines in that they are usually more specific with regard to the airway devices that are suggested at different points in the algorithm. This specificity accounts for usual institutional practices, the availability of particular airway adjuncts, and the familiarity of individual practitioners with different airway management techniques.

One of the most well-studied and commonly cited algorithms is the emergency airway algorithm, developed at the R. Adams Cowley Shock Trauma Center at the University of Maryland.[16] This algorithm is a simplified version of the ASA's DAA and focuses on rapid sequence intubation with up to 3 laryngoscopic attempts (using a bougie, if indicated), followed by an attempt at LMA ventilation, and finally the performance of a surgical airway, if ventilation has not been established. In a 10-year retrospective analysis of the use of this algorithm in more than 30,000 patients, the overall rate of surgical airway was 0.1%, and no patients died of a failed airway.[16]

NONANESTHESIOLOGY SPECIALTIES

Other specialists involved in the management of the airway include critical care physicians, emergency medicine physicians, and otorhinolaryngologists. None of the national societies in the United States for these specialties have their own published guidelines for the management of the difficult airway. The critical care and otorhinolaryngology literature on the difficult airway commonly reference the guidelines and algorithms developed by anesthesia societies.[17,18]

Because these guidelines and algorithms are focused primarily on the elective management of airways in the perioperative setting, several assumptions are made that often do not apply to emergency or prehospital settings. In these circumstances, clinicians may not have the opportunity to perform a detailed assessment of the potential for a difficult airway (owing to the emergent need for intubation); patients may not be cooperative or stable enough to undergo awake intubation; patients are frequently unfasted; and awakening the patients is often not an option (eg, patients in extremis). Therefore, several difficult airway algorithms have been developed for use in the emergency department or prehospital setting. One of the most commonly cited is the algorithm developed by Drs Walls and Murphy, which consists of 4 distinct algorithms for separate scenarios: the main algorithm, the crash airway algorithm (for patients in extremis), the difficult airway algorithm (for the predicted difficult airway), and the failed airway algorithm (for the CICV scenario). The algorithms have been developed by expert opinion and modified several times using the guidelines from the ASA and DAS and a nonsystematic review of the literature as references. These algorithms have many similarities to the anesthesia society algorithms, but they do not focus on awakening patients. One notable difference is the recommendation to administer succinylcholine if the initial attempt at intubation is unsuccessful during a crash airway.

The ASA's DAA itself has also been modified for the trauma setting. The 2003 DAA was modified in 2005 by Wilson,[19] who also developed specific algorithms for various trauma settings. The ASA's Committee on Trauma and Emergency Preparedness has recently updated these modifications using the latest revisions to the DAA.[20] In addition to providing specific recommendations on cricoid pressure, manual in-line stabilization, and VAL in the trauma setting, algorithms are suggested to aid in the management of various difficult airway scenarios, including closed head injury, airway disruption, oral/maxillofacial trauma, cervical spine injury, and airway compression.

FUTURE CONSIDERATIONS/SUMMARY

Despite the number of different practice guidelines available to assist practitioners with the management of a difficult airway, no evidence supports one set of guidelines over another. It is clear, however, that they play an important role in patient safety. Even if not implemented exactly as written, the dissemination of these guidelines encourages airway practitioners to consider their strategies and formulate specific plans for the management of a predicted or unexpected difficult airway.

The different algorithms and guidelines are highly variable owing to the lack of an optimal technologic solution for all difficult airway scenarios. The continued proliferation of airway devices designed to aid the management of the difficult airway has the potential to improve outcomes but may leave the airway practitioner with unanswered questions regarding which device to use in which circumstance. Each device has unique properties that may be advantageous in certain situations, yet limiting in others. Specific airway management techniques are greatly influenced by individual disease and anatomy, and successful management may require a combination of devices and techniques. It is important, therefore, that practitioners develop their own individual strategies, founded on their own clinical experience and skills, and that any technique chosen is well rehearsed in patients with nonproblematic airways before it is implemented in those who are likely to be difficult.

No evidence exists to support one set of guidelines over another as a gold standard. Further research is necessary to compare differing aspects of the various guidelines and algorithms to determine which recommendations may be applicable to a wide spectrum of practitioners and which may be considered standards of care. Currently, there is consensus on several aspects of difficult airway management, including the importance of a preemptive airway assessment when feasible, a requirement for the development of skill with advanced airway techniques, and the need for a preplanned airway management strategy that culminates with surgical airway access in the CICV scenario.

REFERENCES

1. Claassen JA. The gold standard: not a golden standard. BMJ 2005;330(7500): 1121.
2. Timmermans S, Berg M. The gold standard: the challenge of evidence-based medicine and standardization in health care. Philadelphia: Temple University Press; 2003.
3. Versi E. "Gold standard" is an appropriate term. BMJ 1992;305(6846):187.
4. Caplan RA, Posner KL, Ward RJ, et al. Adverse respiratory events in anesthesia: a closed claims analysis. Anesthesiology 1990;72(5):828–33.
5. Practice guidelines for management of the difficult airway. A report by the American Society of Anesthesiologists Task Force on Management of the Difficult Airway. Anesthesiology 1993;78(3):597–602.
6. Apfelbaum JL, Hagberg CA, Caplan RA, et al. Practice guidelines for management of the difficult airway: an updated report by the American Society of Anesthesiologists Task Force on Management of the Difficult Airway. Anesthesiology 2013;118(2):251–70.
7. Caplan RA, Apfelbaum JL, Connis RT, et al. In reply. Anesthesiology 2013;119(3): 733.
8. Chrimes N, Fritz P. The vortex approach: management of the unanticipated difficult airway. Los Gatos (CA): Smashwords; 2013.
9. Levine AI, DeMaria S Jr. An updated report by the American Society of Anesthesiologists Task Force on Management of the Difficult Airway: where is the aspiration risk assessment? Anesthesiology 2013;119(3):731–2.
10. Henderson JJ, Popat MT, Latto IP, et al. Difficult Airway Society guidelines for management of the unanticipated difficult intubation. Anaesthesia 2004;59(7): 675–94.
11. Law JA, Broemling N, Cooper RM, et al. The difficult airway with recommendations for management – part 1 – difficult tracheal intubation encountered in an unconscious/induced patient. Can J Anaesth 2013;60(11):1089–118.
12. Langeron O, Bourgain JL, Laccoureye O, et al. Difficult airway algorithms and management. Ann Fr Anesth Reanim 2008;27(1):41–5.
13. Braun U, Goldmann K, Hempel V, et al. Airway management: Leitlinie der Deutschen Gesellschaft für Anästhesiologie und Intensivmedizin. Anästhesiol Intensivmed 2004;45:302–6.

14. Petrini F, Accorsi A, Adrario E, et al. Recommendations for airway control and difficult airway management. Minerva Anestesiol 2005;71(11):617–57.
15. Metzner J, Posner KL, Lam MS, et al. Closed claims' analysis. Best Pract Res Clin Anaesthesiol 2011;25(2):263–76.
16. Stephens CT, Kahntroff S, Dutton RP. The success of emergency endotracheal intubation in trauma patients: a 10-year experience at a major adult trauma referral center. Anesth Analg 2009;109(3):866–72.
17. Lavery GG, McCloskey BV. The difficult airway in adult critical care. Crit Care Med 2008;36(7):2163–73.
18. Mark L, Herzer K, Akst S, et al. General considerations of anesthesia and difficult airway management. In: Flint PW, Haughey BH, Lund VJ, et al, editors. Cummings otolaryngology – head and neck surgery. 5th edition. Philadelphia: Mosby Elsevier; 2010. p. 108–20.
19. Wilson WC. Trauma: airway management. ASA Newsl 2005;69(11):9–16.
20. Hagberg CA, Kaslow O. Difficult airway management algorithm in trauma updated by COTEP. ASA Newsl 2014;78(9):56–60.

Strengths and Limitations of Airway Techniques

Richard M. Cooper, MSc, MD, FRCPC[a,b],*

KEYWORDS

- Airway management • Laryngoscopy • Tracheal intubation • Video laryngoscopy
- Supraglottic airways • Tracheal extubation • Complications • Extubation

KEY POINTS

- Face mask ventilation and direct laryngoscopy fail in a significant number of patients, in some of whom it is predictable; however, many are not, necessitating transition to a backup plan.
- A supraglottic airway may restore effective oxygenation.
- Fiberoptic and video laryngoscopes (VLs) may provide good laryngeal exposure that is not possible by direct laryngoscopy.
- VLs are available in channeled and nonchanneled configurations.

INTRODUCTION

Until recently, airway management choices were limited; a patient could be managed by face mask ventilation or intubated using direct laryngoscopy. The options available at present are far greater: face mask and supraglottic airway (SGA) devices, tracheal intubation (blindly, via an SGA, using a flexible endoscope, a lightwand, ferromagnetic intubation, direct laryngoscopy, video laryngoscopy, and an optical stylet), and a surgical airway. In addition, extubation strategies should be considered for the patient with a difficult airway. Within each of these categories, there are numerous varieties of devices and techniques. Practice guidelines have been developed by expert committees representing national or specialty societies, recommending strategies to be implemented under specific or general circumstances.[1–4] These guidelines are discussed elsewhere in this article. Unfortunately, few of the recommendations are evidence based and rely largely on expert opinion.[5] Absent such

Disclosure: The author is an unpaid member of the Scientific Advisory Committee of Verathon Medical. He does not have any equity in any company manufacturing airway devices.
[a] Department of Anesthesia, University of Toronto, Toronto, Ontario, Canada; [b] Department of Anesthesia and Pain Management, Toronto General Hospital, 200 Elizabeth Street, 3EN-421, Toronto, Ontario M5G 2C4, Canada
* Department of Anesthesia, University of Toronto, Toronto, Ontario, Canada.
E-mail address: richard.cooper@uhn.ca

Anesthesiology Clin 33 (2015) 241–255
http://dx.doi.org/10.1016/j.anclin.2015.02.006
1932-2275/15/$ – see front matter © 2015 Elsevier Inc. All rights reserved.

Box 2
Examples of supraglottic airways

- LMA (Teleflex, Wayne, PA):
  - LMA Classic (reusable)/Unique (single use), sizes: 1, 1.5, 2, 2.5, 3, 4, 5, 6
  - LMA ProSeal (reusable)/Supreme (single use), sizes: 1, 1.5, 2, 2.5, 3, 4, 5
  - LMA Fastrach (reusable/single use), sizes: 3, 4, 5
  - LMA Flexible (reusable/single use), sizes: 2, 2.5, 3, 4, 5, 6
- I-gel (Intersurgical, Wokingham, Berkshire UK), sizes: 1, 1.5, 2, 2.5, 3, 4, 5
- Laryngeal Tube S and SD (King/Ambu, Noblesville, IN), sizes: 2, 2.5, 3, 4, 5
- Air-Q (Mercury Medical, Clearwater, FL), sizes: 1, 1.5, 2.0, 2.5, 3.5, 4.5

---

surgical procedure.[11] NAP4 studied major airway-related complications, including brain injury, death, an unintended surgical airway, and intensive care unit (ICU) admission as a consequence of an airway event. Presumably these represent the worst outcomes with minor complications occurring with much higher frequency. Events leading to major adverse outcomes included regurgitation (and aspiration), air leaks, trauma, and device displacement. Proper patient and device selection, insertion and fixation techniques, and vigilance during use likely lessen the complications. The NAP4 investigators found that first-generation iSGAs were often used in higher-risk patients with an increased risk of regurgitation, in cases involving predicted difficult airways, during urgent surgery, and in obese patients. Although SGA use has been described for parturient patients, morbidly obese patients, and patients in the prone or lithotomy position, the clinician should recognize that these uses often go beyond the manufacturers' recommendations and may put both patient and clinician in jeopardy. Chapter 11 of the NAP4 document provides an excellent discussion of these points (**Box 3**).[13]

FLEXIBLE ENDOSCOPIC INTUBATION

Flexible endoscopic intubation, long regarded as the gold standard technique in managing difficult intubation, has distinguished itself for its versatility. It can be introduced

---

Box 3
Predictors of difficulty with SGA insertion or ventilation

- Reduced mouth opening
- Supraglottic, extraglottic, glottic, or subglottic pathology
- Fixed cervical spine flexion deformity
- During application of cricoid pressure
- Male gender
- Increased body mass index
- Poor dentition
- Lack of access to airway during use

From Law JA, Broemling N, Cooper RM, et al. The difficult airway with recommendations for management - Part 2 - The anticipated difficult airway. Can J Anaesth 2013;60(11):1123; with permission.

---

through the nose, mouth, or stoma; it can be anteflexed and retroflexed as well as rotated to the right and left. With skill, it is well suited for awake intubation, allowing the patient to maintain spontaneous ventilation, airway patency, and protective reflexes. In many ways, it fails when it is more needed—the unanticipated failed airway with deteriorating oxygen levels. Time is required to obtain and set up the equipment, blood and secretions may obscure the view, and in contrast to the devices and techniques discussed later, the endoscopist may observe the endoscope entering the trachea but advancement of the TT is entirely blind and frequently arytenoid impaction occurs.[14] Nonetheless, facility with this device is an essential skill because there are situations when no other technique short of an invasive airway is likely to succeed. This skill must be practiced to acquire and maintain proficiency.[15] The role of the flexible endoscope is discussed in greater detail elsewhere in this issue.

LARYNGOSCOPY

This airway arena has also become a crowded space. Until recently, choices were limited to minor variations of the Miller (1941) and Macintosh (1943) direct laryngoscope blades.[16] During the past 15 years, there has been a proliferation of new devices using fiberoptic and video chip technology.[17–19] Line-of-sight direct laryngoscopy is limited by the anatomic obstacles that obstruct the view of the vocal cords, such as the maxillary incisors, the size and compliance of the tongue, and the ability to achieve prognathia and when necessary to push the larynx posteriorly. Prediction of a difficult direct laryngoscopy is an inexact science, suffering from poor sensitivity and specificity. A meta-analysis included 35 studies involving 50,760 adult patients deemed appropriate for intubation following anesthesia induction. The studies had to describe the bedside predictors of difficulty used (eg, Mallampati view, thyromental distance, sternomental distance, mouth opening, Wilson risk score, or a combination of tests) and the laryngeal view obtained. A Cormack-Lehane score of 3 or greater indicated difficult (direct) laryngoscopy and occurred in 5.8% of patients.[20] Other investigators, using an Intubation Difficulty Score (IDS) took into consideration the number of required attempts, the number of additional operators, alternative techniques, laryngeal view, excess lifting force, and external laryngeal pressure. An IDS greater than 5 indicated at least a moderately difficult intubation. Although an IDS of zero (no difficulty at all) was encountered in 55% of operating room (OR) intubations, minor difficulties were seen in 37%, a score of greater than 5 was seen in 7.7%, and difficult direct laryngoscopy, requiring 2 or 3 attempts, was seen in 9% of patients.[21] Outcomes are consistently worse when intubations are attempted outside the OR, when the focus is on higher-risk populations or patients with multiple predictors of difficulty.

Investigators have experimented with different positions, including sniffing; neutral, simple extension[22]; and head elevation (flexion-flexion).[23] The combinations of head and neck contortions have probably been exhausted, yet a position that aligns the airway axes has not been identified. When the larynx is more difficult to see, one may attempt intubation blindly, exert more force,[24] make multiple efforts, and frequently resort to approaches that have already proved to be unsuccessful.[25] Esophageal intubation is more likely, potentially distending the stomach, increasing the risk of regurgitation, and delaying oxygenation. Multiple attempts are associated with an increased risk of complications.[26,27]

NAP4 and other studies indicate that airway difficulties increase with increasing patient size, a problem projected to continue at an alarming pace. Alternatives to achieving a direct line of sight have to be found.

Originally, coherent fiberoptic bundles incorporated into an anatomically shaped retraction blade made vocal cord viewing possible in many patients for whom successful direct laryngoscopy could not be achieved. These devices include the Bullard (Olympus), UpsherScope (Mercury Medical), and WuScope (Achi Wu) laryngoscopes; they were challenging to learn, cumbersome to use, and costly to acquire. Although these devices still have their proponents, they are no longer manufactured.[6,18] Fiberoptic stylets include the Bonfils (Karl Storz), Shikani SOS, and Levitan FPS (Clarus Medical). These devices can be used alone or in conjunction with direct laryngoscopy. When miniature video cameras, primarily complementary metal oxide semiconductors, were embedded into modified laryngoscope blades, the devices were familiar, were portable, facilitated simultaneous observing by multiple people, and found a variety of clinical applications. These devices include among others the GlideScope (Verathon), McGrath (Aircraft Medical), the C-MAC (Karl Storz), Airtraq (Prodol), AWS100 (Ambu), King Vision scope (Ambu), and TruView PCD (Truphatek).

VLs are classified as channeled versus nonchanneled or Macintosh-style curve versus exaggerated angulation of the blade. Both these characteristics have implications with respect to how (and when) they are used and the advantages or limitations they impose (**Box 4**).

Channeled Devices

All channeled devices use blades that are more angulated than those of the Macintosh-style laryngoscopes.

These VLs have a channel integrated into the blade meant to facilitate easier TT advancement. Examples of such devices include Airway Scope AWS100 (Ambu/Pentax)

Box 4
Alternatives to direct laryngoscopy

- Rigid fiberoptic laryngoscopes
  - WuScope
  - UpsherScope Ultra
  - Bullard Elite (Gyrus ACMI, Southborough, MA)
- Channeled video laryngoscopes
  - Airway Scope100 (Ambu, Ballerup, Denmark)
  - Airtraq and Airtraq Avant (Prodol Meditec, Vizcaya, Spain)
  - King Vision scope—channeled blade (King/Ambu)
- Nonchanneled video laryngoscopes
  - Macintosh style
    - C-MAC (Karl Storz, Tuttlingen, Germany)
    - GlideScope Direct and LoPro reusable and single-use T-MAC (Verathon, Bothel, WA)
    - McGrath MAC (Aircraft Medical, Edinburgh, UK)
  - Angulated blades
    - C-MAC D-blade (Karl Storz)
    - GlideScope reusable: LoPro Titanium and GVL; single use: LoPro SU (Verathon)
    - McGrath Series5 and McGrath D-blade (Aircraft Medical)
    - EVO2/Truview PCD (Truphatek, Netanya, Israel)

and Airtraq and the newer Airtraq Avant (Prodol). The King Vision scope is available in both channeled and nonchanneled configurations. A TT is preloaded, and both the VL and the TT are advanced as a unit. All these devices have reusable and single-use components (with the exception of the original Airtraq) and are described briefly. More complete descriptions are found elsewhere.[6,17,19]

Ambu airway scope (AWS100)

The AWS100 consists of a portable flexible video baton connected to a 2.4-inch liquid-crystal display (LCD) monitor. The single-use polycarbonate PBlade is available in 1 size, and its channel, along the right side of the blade, can accommodate endotracheal tubes corresponding to an internal diameter (ID) of 6.5 to 8.0 mm. The technique requires direct elevation of the epiglottis to successfully advance the tube. There is a composite video signal port to enable image capture.

When this technique was initially conceived, cervical stabilization was a priority. A summary of the clinical studies may be found elsewhere.[6,19] Like in all channeled laryngoscopes, the blades are bulkier than those of nonchanneled devices (height 18 mm), which restricts its use to patients with a normal mouth opening. In addition, the length of the blade and handle makes insertion difficult in patients with large breasts or hyperinflated lungs. Elevation of the epiglottis and susceptibility to fogging remain additional potential problems.

Airtraq

The Airtraq is technically an optical laryngoscope in that the image is acquired via plastic prisms and lenses. The original version, entirely disposable and available in 7 different single-use configurations, has been modified, lowering its cost. The new Airtraq Avant consists of a reusable optical element with single-use clear plastic blades. It is available in only 2 adult sizes (for TT ID 6–7.5 mm and 7.0–8.5 mm). The user may choose to obtain the view via the eyepiece or by an optional propriety camera. Two other options have become available for viewing and recording: a Wi-Fi camera with an integrated LCD monitor and a simple adapter for viewing on an iPhone or iPad. Midline insertion is recommended, and it can be placed either anterior or posterior to the epiglottis.

The Airtraq does not require a capital investment, but the cost per use of the original model was difficult to justify for routine use. The Avant version is a fraction of that cost, but currently, it is available in only 2 adult sizes or oral intubation. The technique is easily learned and effective in a variety of challenging situations.[6,19] Laryngeal exposure is good, but the image quality cannot compare with other devices in its class.

King Vision scope

The King Vision scope has been redesigned. The older version consisted of a 2.4-in VGA (video graphics array) reusable OLED (organic light emitting diode) display and a single-use, single adult-size polycarbonate blade. There is a video-output port that accepts the yellow (video) jack of a conventional RCA plug. Three AAA batteries are housed in the handle. The older blade incorporates a light-emitting diode (LED) light source and a video chip, both of which are discarded after use. By placing the light source and camera into a reusable video baton, only the clear plastic blade cover is discarded. Both the new and old versions are available in channeled and nonchanneled configurations. As of this writing, there are no published reports in human subjects with either version. The author assumes interchangeability of the original and newer versions. Here the channeled version is discussed.

The channeled blade is thicker, with a blade height of 18 mm (compared with 13 mm for its nonchanneled counterpart). Like the other channeled blades, the TT is positioned in the channel guide before insertion into the patient's mouth. With the head in a neutral position, midline placement in the mouth is recommended. The blade is advanced around the tongue base and positioned in the vallecula. The TT is advanced taking care that its trajectory is appropriate. All the channeled blades have this in common: TT advancement is achieved by manipulation of the laryngoscope in 2 planes, side to side and rocking forward or backward. Some regard this as an advantage; others view it as a limitation, preferring independent manipulation of the laryngoscope and the TT.

The thickness of the blade, particularly the channeled one, and the length of the blade-monitor assembly may create a challenge in introducing it in the mouth of patients with small mouth opening, a big chest, or reduced atlantoaxial extension.

Nonchanneled Devices

The nonchanneled devices are divided into 2 categories, Macintosh-style laryngoscopes and angulated blades, both having video cameras embedded into the distal blade.

Macintosh Style

The devices and the technique recommended are familiar to laryngoscopists. Patients are ordinarily in the sniffing position. The blade is introduced along the right side of the tongue and is displaced leftward. A TT stylet is considered optional. The view may be obtained directly or by observing a monitor. This view is often more revealing than what is seen when looking directly into the patient's mouth, but not dramatically so. Often, external laryngeal manipulation or use of a bougie is required.[28–31] An improved view is a consequence of the more distal location of the video camera and a visual field wider than that possible with line of sight. The biggest advantage of these devices is their familiarity, their utility both directly and indirectly, and the display that can be viewed by more than just the operator, thereby facilitating instruction and participation. The disadvantage is the limited improvement over direct laryngoscopy (DL) they afford.

C-MAC

This device from Karl Storz has gone through several iterations from the DCI to the V-MAC and more recently the C-MAC.[6,17] Although discussion is restricted to the current product, performance does not seem to be dramatically different. The C-MAC system consists of an electronic module linked by means of a cable to a proprietary monitor. The electronic module can be plugged into several styles and sizes of blades (Miller, Macintosh, or D-blade, discussed later). Snapshot or video recordings can be initiated by activating a button on the handle or the monitor and stored onto a Secure Digital card or transferred to a Universal Serial Bus flash drive.

McGrath MAC

This Macintosh-style VL from Aircraft Medical is (as of this writing) available in a single adult size and consists of a rigid CameraStick with a 2.5-in portrait-oriented LCD monitor attached to the handle. It uses a proprietary battery housed in its handle, with its life expectancy digitally displayed on the monitor. The laryngoscope handle, monitor, and camera stick are immersible for high-level disinfection. Its vertical height is 11.9 mm where the camera stick meets a single-use polycarbonate Macintosh blade, clipped in place over the camera stick. Although the LCD screen is visible to more than the operator, it is small and the device lacks a video output, making recording difficult.

There are numerous testimonials but, as of this writing, no published reports of its performance. The technique recommended by the manufacturer is identical to that used for DL, with or without a stylet, obtaining the view directly or indirectly on the monitor. How similar these views are is speculative until comparisons are published, but the device is lightweight, free of wires, familiar, and inexpensive. Two other McGrath devices are discussed later.

GlideScope MAC

In addition to the GlideScope Direct (size 3.5), Verathon has added the LoPro Glide-Scope Macintosh-style blades (sizes 3 and 4 in both reusable titanium and single-use plastic). The lower-profile laryngoscope is lightweight, with a maximum vertical profile of 11 mm at the camera and LED light source. The camera lens is heated to prevent fogging. The newer AVL monitor has recording capability for snapshots and videos. The monitor has a new file management and video replay feature to facilitate teaching and clinical review. In addition, there is a video output to enable an external display or image capture. Like the McGrath MAC, there are encouraging testimonials but as of this writing, no published reports assessing its performance.

The manufacturer recommends that both the Direct and LoPro-MACs be used like a conventional Macintosh laryngoscope. The operator can choose either direct or video view, with or without a stylet; however, by design, the indirect view with the LoPro-MAC is likely to be significantly better than the direct view due to the orientation of the camera. This difference seems greater than that encountered with other Macintosh VLs, but this requires verification. In contrast to the GlideScope Direct, intended primarily as a DL trainer, the role of the LoPro MAC remains to be determined.

Angulated Blades

Unlike the Macintosh-style VLs, these devices do not provide a useful direct view because the distal location of the video camera and the angulation of the blade result in a more anteriorly orientated image; this provides superior laryngeal imaging in many patients in whom a line of sight cannot be achieved but it requires that the laryngoscopist be able to deliver and advance the TT to an object he/she cannot see directly.[32] For example, in an early study using the GlideScope, a good or excellent laryngeal view was obtained in 99% of 722 patients, many of whom had features predictive of difficulty had DL been used; intubation failed in 3.7% of patients, half of whom had a Cormack-Lehane grade I view.[33] Delivery and TT advancement are techniques that can be acquired.

What follows is a general description of the technique, common to all these devices. Patient positioning is less important because it is unnecessary to align the anatomic axes; optical alignment is achieved by the video camera. The author generally uses the neutral position to facilitate insertion of the blade into the patient's mouth. In the sniffing position, the laryngoscope handle may abut on the hand of the person performing cricoid pressure or the chest of the patient. Next, the laryngoscope is introduced in the midline. The tongue does not have to be displaced leftward, but the blade must be smoothly advanced to the tongue base. The author recommends the use of a film of water-soluble lubricant on the blade surface. Commonly, the laryngoscope is inserted too deeply and this is not noticed, leading to several undesirable things:

- The axis of the larynx may be deflected upward, increasing the angle of incidence with the VL[32]; this may result in greater laryngeal exposure but at the expense of a more difficult intubation.
- It narrows the visual field; a wider view is more desirable.
- It increases the area of the blind spot and may increase the risk of a soft-tissue injury.[34] The blind spot is the space between the lips and the camera. The use of a properly inserted stylet, recessed within the TT, is not the cause of this injury. These complications are entirely avoidable if the operator directly

observes the advancement of the TT as it passes from the lips, past the soft palate.

- The epiglottis may be inadvertently downfolded and pushed into the laryngeal inlet.[35]

To avoid multiple laryngoscopies, the first attempt should be optimal and a stylet should be used whenever an angulated VL is used. Neither the type of stylet nor the precise shape is as important as the technique. The types of stylets available include the malleable, rigid, dynamic, and optical. A malleable stylet can be a tracheal introducer, for example, Mallinckrodt Satin-Slip intubating stylet, Frova Introducer (Cook), and an Eschmann-type bougie; the GlideRite (Verathon) is an example of a rigid stylet; the Parker Flex-It (Parker Medical) and the Truflex (Truphatek) are examples of dynamic stylets in that anteflexion can be performed during laryngoscopy; an example of an optical stylet is the flexible bronchoscope.[36] The larynx is viewed using the VL, and the bronchoscope is used to redirect the tube into the trachea.

In patients with a small mouth opening, it is sometimes helpful to introduce the TT before the VL. In addition, selection of a lower-profile laryngoscope is desirable. The laryngoscopist should deliberately identify the uvula and epiglottis, avoiding excessively deep insertion. An attempt should be made to hold the VL so that the vocal cords are vertically oriented. With most devices, the VL blade should be inserted into the vallecula. The direction (but not the amount) of the lifting force is similar to that required for DL, thereby creating space in the oropharynx. The styletted TT is carefully inserted into the mouth, close to the laryngoscope blade and closely apposed to the tongue. The tube is then elevated as if to further retract the tongue and gently directed toward the glottic chink with a simple tilt.

Advancement of the tube may require rotation to disengage its tip from the anterior tracheal wall. It should fall into the airway with no force being required. Although not discussed, these devices are also appropriate for nasal intubation.

In general, the angulated blades provide better laryngeal exposure but may present the operator with a challenge in delivering and advancing the TT, resulting in frustration, defeat, or recognition of an opportunity for significant clinical advantages. Longer intubation times may be encountered, although this may not apply to patients with more difficult airways. The strategies described are applicable to the EVO, Glide-Scope, McGrath Series5, and C-MAC D-blade mentioned later.

EVO/Truview/PCD
When originally introduced, the device consisted of an angulated Macintosh-style blade with a 45° hoptical lens on the undersurface of the blade. Subsequently, a digital camera mount became available, providing a larger LCD display and simplifying recording. The current iteration is the PCD, which couples a video camera to the optical lens and a dedicated LCD display. There are few studies describing these laryngoscopes, and most are small, involve normal airways, and pertain to pediatrics.

King Vision nonchanneled
The King Vision scope was described earlier. The blade is available in both channeled and nonchanneled configurations. The nonchanneled blade has a slimmer 13-mm profile and requires the use of a stylet. As of this writing, there are no studies comparing the 2 versions or clinical evaluations performed on human subjects.

GlideScope: GVL and LoPro single use and reusable
Since its introduction in 2001, the GlideScope has retained the essential shape of the blade with a fairly acute 60° angulation. GlideScopes are available in 4 configurations

and in a wide range of sizes, as single-use or reusable devices. Single-use blades use a video baton with disposable clear plastic blades (Stat) or the newer lower-profile blades that mimic the reusable titanium models. They range in size from 0 to 5 (although these do not correspond to conventional sizing) and are suitable for neonates to large adults. For comparison purposes, the size 4 single-use blades have heights of 16 and 11 mm in the original baton/Stat and newer LoPro configurations, respectively. The reusable blades are either plastic or titanium, with corresponding vertical profiles of 14 and 11 mm, respectively. As mentioned earlier, this has consistently provided laryngeal exposure but created some challenges in the delivery and advancement of the TT.[32]

There is a considerable volume of literature relating to the GlideScope in normal and challenging airways, in operating rooms, in emergency departments, in ICUs, and by prehospital responders. A review of this literature is beyond the scope of this article and can be found elsewhere.[2,6,19,37,38]

McGrath Series5/McGrath X-blade (angled blade)

This device was the first VL from Aircraft Medical. It is a lightweight, battery-operated device with an adjustable camera stick that can be retracted or extended to 3 different adult lengths. This device is covered by a single-use, 60° angulated 13-mm polycarbonate blade, shaped similarly to the GlideScope. The image is displayed on a 1.7-in LCD monitor mounted atop the handle.

Laryngeal exposure and image quality are good. Clinical performance, although less well studied than that of the GlideScope, has been favorable in patients with normal airway anatomy, anticipated difficult or failed direct laryngoscopy. It has no video output or recording capability and is susceptible to fogging. The battery life and camera stick have been problematic, resulting in the later development of the McGrath MAC with its fixed camera stick and improved proprietary battery. More recently, Aircraft Medical as introduced the McGrath X-blade, which is a single-use polycarbonate blade cover with an angulated design similar to the Series5. As yet, there are no published reports regarding its utility. A particularly compelling aspect of the McGrath entry is price; the manufacturer has priced the products in a manner that lowers to barrier to adoption of VL for routine use.

C-MAC with D-blade

The Karl Storz C-MAC, described earlier, resulted in a significant improvement compared with DL; however, a significant number of patients still required external laryngeal pressure and the use of a gum elastic bougie,[31,39] prompting the introduction of an angulated blade, shaped like a half-moon and known as the D-blade (for difficult or Doerges, one of its developers).[40] The D-blade is compatible with the electronic module and monitor; it can also be used with a stand-alone portable monitor that sits atop the handle.

Like the other angulated blades, direct viewing is not advised with the D-blade and a stylet and midline insertion are recommended. In a small study of patients with (presumed or encountered) difficult airways, the D-blade and GlideScope produced similar outcomes, both outperforming DL with respect to laryngoscopic views and first attempt success.[41]

EXTUBATION

Evidence indicates the lack of progress in reducing injuries following extubation.[42] Identification of patients at increased risk and appropriate strategies to increase the need for or safety of reintubation has been discussed.[43–45]

Airway exchange catheters are commercially available and can be used to maintain airway access following extubation, to serve as a stylet to facilitate reintubation[46] or a conduit for the supplementation of oxygen. Oxygen supplementation by insufflation, positive pressure, or jet ventilation should be done with great caution as serious complications have been reported.[47] If insufflation is used, only low-flows (eg, 1–2 liters/minute) should be used; with positive pressure and jet ventilation, every effort should be made to minimize obstruction with delivery of only enough oxygen to forestall life-threatening hypoxemia. Reintubation with an exchange catheter is greatly facilitated by minimizing the disparity between the inner and outer diameters of the TT and exchange catheters, respectively. Use of a VL as a tongue retractor and a means of visualizing the reintubation is highly recommended.[48]

SUMMARY

During the past 25 years, there have been major developments in airway management devices. These devices should be incorporated into successful strategies. These devices can be used effectively only if used regularly. Focus should be maintained on the essential goal of airway management, maintaining oxygenation, and not compromising this objective by persisting with ineffective approaches. Because one cannot always predict the success of the methods chosen, one cannot become overly confident about any single method; this may involve moving beyond the face mask to an SGA or from DL to VL (or vice versa). There will always be patients in whom flexible endoscopy is the most appropriate approach, and one cannot afford to abandon this essential skill. Help, when possible, should be summoned early and consideration given to awakening the patient, if that option is possible. If these approaches fail, an invasive airway may be required. Extubation is always elective; a strategy that maximizes the probability of achieving reintubation should always be considered in the patient with a difficult airway.

REFERENCES

1. Apfelbaum JL, Hagberg CA, Caplan RA, et al. Practice guidelines for management of the difficult airway: an updated report by the American society of anesthesiologists task force on management of the difficult airway. Anesthesiology 2013;118(2):251–70.
2. Law JA, Broemling N, Cooper RM, et al. The difficult airway with recommendations for management - Part 1-Difficult tracheal intubation encountered in an unconscious/induced patient. Can J Anaesth 2013;60(11):1089–118.
3. Law JA, Broemling N, Cooper RM, et al. The difficult airway with recommendations for management - Part 2-The anticipated difficult airway. Can J Anaesth 2013;60(11):1119–38.
4. Henderson JJ, Popat MT, Latto IP, et al. Difficult Airway Society guidelines for management of the unanticipated difficult intubation. Anaesthesia 2004;59(7): 675–94.
5. Crosby ET. An evidence-based approach to airway management: is there a role for clinical practice guidelines? Anaesthesia 2011;66:112–8.
6. Cooper RM, Law JA. Rigid fiberoptic and video laryngoscopes. In: Hung O, Murphy MF, editors. Management of the difficult and failed airway. 2nd edition. New York: McGraw Hill; 2011. p. 159–85.
7. Verghese C, Mena G, Ferson D, et al. Laryngeal mask airway. In: Hagberg CA, editor. Benumof and Hagberg's airway management. 3rd edition. Philadelphia: Elsevier Saunders; 2013. p. 443–65.

8. Cook T. Non-laryngeal mask airway supraglottic airway devices. In: Hagberg C, editor. Benumof and Hagberg's airway management. 3rd edition. Philadelphia: Elsevier Saunders; 2013. p. 466–507.

9. Weingart SD. Preoxygenation, reoxygenation, and delayed sequence intubation in the emergency department. J Emerg Med 2011;40(6):661–7.

10. Langeron O, Masso E, Huraux C, et al. Prediction of difficult mask ventilation. Anesthesiology 2000;92(5):1229–36.

11. Ramachandran SK, Mathis MR, Tremper KK, et al. Predictors and clinical outcomes from failed Laryngeal Mask Airway Unique™: a study of 15,795 patients. Anesthesiology 2012;116:1217–26.

12. van Zundert TC, Brimacombe JR, Ferson DZ, et al. Archie Brain: celebrating 30 years of development in laryngeal mask airways. Anaesthesia 2012;67(12): 1375–85.

13. Cook TM, Woodall N, Frerk C. Fourth National Audit Project of the Royal College of Anaesthetists and Difficult Airway Society. Major complications of airway management in the United Kingdom. Report and Findings. London, 2011. Available at: http://www.rcoa.ac.uk/nap4.

14. Johnson DM, From AM, Smith RB, et al. Endoscopic study of mechanisms of failure of endotracheal tube advancement into the trachea during awake fiberoptic orotracheal intubation. Anesthesiology 2005;102(5):910–4.

15. Heidegger T. Airway management: standardization, simplicity, and daily practice are the keys to success. Anesth Analg 2010;111(4):1073 [author reply: 4].

16. Levitan RM, Hagberg CA. Upper airway retraction: new and old laryngoscope blades. In: Hagberg CA, editor. Benumof and Hagberg's airway management. 3rd edition. Philadelphia: Elsevier Saunders; 2013. p. 508–35.

17. Cavus E, Dorges V. Video laryngoscopes. In: Hagberg CA, editor. Benumof and Hagberg's airway management. Philadelphia: Elsevier Saunders; 2013. p. 536–48.

18. Cooper RM. The role of rigid fiberoptic laryngoscopes. In: Glick DB, Cooper RM, Ovassapian A, editors. The difficult airway: an atlas of tools and techniques for clinical management. New York: Springer; 2013. p. 65–76.

19. Cooper RM, Lee C. Role of rigid video laryngoscopy. In: Glick D, Cooper R, Ovassapian A, editors. The difficult airway: an atlas of tools and techniques for clinical management. New York: Springer; 2013. p. 77–111.

20. Shiga T, Wajima Z, Inoue T, et al. Predicting difficult intubation in apparently normal patients: a meta-analysis of bedside screening test performance. Anesthesiology 2005;103(2):429–37.

21. Adnet F, Racine SX, Borron SW, et al. A survey of tracheal intubation difficulty in the operating room: a prospective observational study. Acta Anaesthesiol Scand 2001;45(3):327–32.

22. Adnet F, Baillard C, Borron SW, et al. Randomized study comparing the "sniffing position" with simple head extension for laryngoscopic view in elective surgery patients. Anesthesiology 2001;95(4):836–41.

23. Levitan RM, Mechem CC, Ochroch EA, et al. Head-elevated laryngoscopy position: improving laryngeal exposure during laryngoscopy by increasing head elevation. Ann Emerg Med 2003;41(3):322–30.

24. Santoni BG, Hindman BJ, Puttlitz CM, et al. Manual in-line stabilization increases pressures applied by the laryngoscope blade during direct laryngoscopy and orotracheal intubation. Anesthesiology 2009;110(1):24–31.

25. Rose DK, Cohen MM. The airway: problems and predictions in 18,500 patients. Can J Aging 1994;41(5 Pt 1):372–83.

26. Mort TC. Emergency tracheal intubation: complications associated with repeated laryngoscopic attempts. Anesth Analg 2004;99(2):607–13.
27. Sakles JC, Chiu S, Mosier J, et al. The importance of first pass success when performing orotracheal intubation in the emergency department. Acad Emerg Med 2013;20(1):71–8.
28. Kaplan MB, Berci G. Videolaryngoscopy in the management of the difficult airway. Can J Anaesth 2004;51(1):94.
29. Cavus E, Thee C, Moeller T, et al. A randomised, controlled crossover comparison of the C-MAC videolaryngoscope with direct laryngoscopy in 150 patients during routine induction of anaesthesia. BMC Anesthesiol 2011;11(1):6.
30. Kaplan MB, Hagberg CA, Ward DS, et al. Comparison of direct and video-assisted views of the larynx during routine intubation. J Clin Anesth 2006;18(5):357–62.
31. Serocki G, Bein B, Scholz J, et al. Management of the predicted difficult airway: a comparison of conventional blade laryngoscopy with video-assisted blade laryngoscopy and the GlideScope. Eur J Anaesthesiol 2010;27(1):24–30 [Miscellaneous Article].
32. Levitan RM, Heitz JW, Sweeney M, et al. The complexities of tracheal intubation with direct laryngoscopy and alternative intubation devices. Ann Emerg Med 2011;57(3):240–7.
33. Cooper RM, Pacey JA, Bishop MJ, et al. Early clinical experience with a new videolaryngoscope (GlideScope). Can J Anaesth 2005;52(2):191–8.
34. Cooper RM. Complications associated with the use of the GlideScope videolaryngoscope. Can J Anaesth 2007;54(1):54–7.
35. van Zundert A, van Zundert T, Brimacombe J. Downfolding of the epiglottis during intubation. Anesth Analg 2010;110(4):1246–7.
36. Doyle DJ. GlideScope-assisted fiberoptic intubation: a new airway teaching method. Anesthesiology 2004;101(5):1252.
37. Paolini JB, Donati F, Drolet P. Review article: video-laryngoscopy: another tool for difficult intubation or a new paradigm in airway management? Can J Anaesth 2013;60(2):184–91.
38. Almarakbi WA, Alhashemi JA, Kaki AM. Adding a conduit to GlideScope blade facilitates tracheal intubation. Prospective randomized study. Saudi Med J 2012;33(6):617–21.
39. Cavus EM, Kieckhaefer JM, Doerges VM, et al. The C-MAC videolaryngoscope: first experiences with a new device for videolaryngoscopy-guided intubation. Anesth Analg 2010;110:473–7 [article].
40. Cavus E, Neumann T, Doerges V, et al. First clinical evaluation of the C-MAC D-Blade videolaryngoscope during routine and difficult intubation. Anesth Analg 2011;112(2):382–5.
41. Serocki G, Neumann T, Scharf E, et al. Indirect videolaryngoscopy with C-MAC D-blade and GlideScope: a randomized, controlled comparison in patients with suspected difficult airways. Minerva Anestesiol 2012;79(2):121–9.
42. Peterson GN, Domino KB, Caplan RA, et al. Management of the difficult airway: a closed claims analysis. Anesthesiology 2005;103(1):33–9.
43. Popat M, Mitchell V, Dravid R, et al. Difficult airway society guidelines for the management of tracheal extubation. Anaesthesia 2012;67(3):318–40.
44. Cavallone LF, Vannucci A. Review article: extubation of the difficult airway and extubation failure. Anesth Analg 2013;116(2):368–83.
45. Cooper RM, Khan SM. Extubation and reintubation of the difficult airway. In: Hagberg C, editor. Benumof and Hagberg's airway management. 3rd edition. Philadelphia: Elsevier-Saunders; 2012. p. 1018–46.

46. Mort TC. Continuous airway access for the difficult extubation: the efficacy of the airway exchange catheter. Anesth Analg 2007;105(5):1357–62.
47. Duggan LV, Law JA, Murphy MF. Brief review: supplementing oxygen through an airway exchange catheter: efficacy, complications, and recommendations. Can J Anaesth 2011;58(6):560–8.
48. Mort TC. Tracheal tube exchange: feasibility of continuous glottic viewing with advanced laryngoscopy assistance. Anesth Analg 2009;108(4):1228–31.

Assessment Before Airway Management

Paul Baker, MBChB, MD, FANZCA

KEYWORDS

- Airway management • Assessment • Techniques • Laryngoscopy • Airway
- Intubation • Tracheal

KEY POINTS

- The techniques and measurements used to predict airway management difficulty are inaccurate. Bedside tests, such as the modified Mallampati test, thyromental distance measurement, sternomental distance measurement and mouth opening, lack accuracy as stand-alone tests to predict difficult tracheal intubation.
- Combining bedside tests and examining multiple physical features improves the chances of predicting a difficult airway but not enough to perform as reliable predictive tests.
- Several studies have examined risk factors associated with airway management techniques and patient factors. This information can be useful when planning to manage a patient's airway.
- It is wise to plan for the unexpected difficult airway: only 50% of difficult airways are anticipated preoperatively.

INTRODUCTION

"An anaesthetist must assess the patient before anaesthesia and devise an appropriate plan of anaesthetic management" – The Good Anaesthetist, Royal College of Anaesthetists 2010.[1]

Airway assessment includes taking a history, performing a physical examination, reviewing the clinical records and performing additional tests. Based on the information gleaned from the airway assessment, a strategy should emerge to cope with each aspect of the patient's airway. This strategy should include options to postpone the case or manage the patient's airway awake and should provide backup plans to deal with failure. Successful identification of physical features that are suggestive of a difficult airway should direct planning toward safe airway management. Accordingly,

Disclosure: Dr P. Baker has received airway management equipment for teaching and research purposes from several companies, including Olympus, Karl Storz, Covidien, LMA, Ambu, Parker, Welch Allyn, Cook, King Systems, Verathon, and Truphatek. He also owns Airway Simulation Limited, which manufactures the ORSIM bronchoscopy simulator.
Department of Anaesthesiology, University of Auckland, Level 12, Room 081, Auckland Support Building 599, Park Road, Grafton, Private Bag 92019, Auckland 1142, New Zealand
E-mail address: paul@airwayskills.co.nz

Anesthesiology Clin 33 (2015) 257–278
http://dx.doi.org/10.1016/j.anclin.2015.02.001
1932-2275/15/$ – see front matter © 2015 Elsevier Inc. All rights reserved.

anesthesiology.theclinics.com

many national airway guidelines emphasize the importance of a thorough and skilled assessment of all patients undergoing anesthesia.[2–4]

Since the original case series describing physical features associated with difficult direct laryngoscopy and difficult tracheal intubation (DTI),[5] several upper airway diagnostic screening tests have been proposed.[6] The latest recommendations from the Canadian Airway Focus Group (CAFG) promote airway assessment at multiple levels, including not only tracheal intubation but also bag mask ventilation, supraglottic airway ventilation, and percutaneous emergency airway access. **Boxes 1–5** have been reproduced from that group and include bedside airway tests and risk factors for airway difficulty.[3]

Many of the airway tests were specifically designed to identify patients without obvious airway pathology or abnormal anatomy who might be harboring a difficult airway. Most of the airway tests can be performed at the bedside in seconds.

Bedside airway tests have been criticized for their poor predictive capability as seen in **Table 1**. This poor predictive capability relates to the low incidence of airway difficulty. In this situation, the positive and negative predictive values will always be low for any test unless their sensitivities and specificities approach 100% (**Fig. 1**).[40]

Other reasons for the poor test performances include a lack of standardized methodology, ill-defined end points, and reliance on subjective assessment, thereby decreasing reproducibility. Most of the tests show only fair interobserver reliability.[49] Predictive tests have also been criticized for relating their findings to the sample from which the study was derived rather than validating the test from a separate population.[14] Subsequent validation studies often find inferior predictive value.[50] Several recent studies have focused on improving the predictive value of airway examination by improving test methodology or combining tests into composite scores.

DEFINITIONS AND INCIDENCE OF AIRWAY DIFFICULTY

One of the problems of finding reliable predictors of a difficult airway concerns a failure to standardize definitions of airway difficulty.[51] Variations in definitions create problems when trying to compare studies of complications and risk factors. A current list of definitions can be found in the CAFG special article, including definitions for

---

Box 1
Predictors of difficult direct laryngoscopy[7–22]

- Limited mouth opening
- Limited mandibular protrusion
- Narrow dental arch
- Decreased thyromental distance
- Modified Mallampati class 3 or 4
- Decreased submandibular compliance
- Decreased sternomental distance
- Limited head and upper neck extension
- Increased neck circumference

From Law AJ, Broemling N, Cooper RM, et al. The difficult airway with recommendations for management-part 2-the anticipated difficult airway. Can J Anaesth 2013;60:1119–38; with permission.

Box 2
Predictors of difficulty in the use of the GlideScope (Verathon Inc, Bothell, WA)[23,24]

Predictors of difficult GlideScope use

- Cormack Lehane grade 3 or 4 view at direct laryngoscopy
- Abnormal neck anatomy, including radiation changes, neck scar, neck pathology, and thick neck
- Limited mandibular protrusion
- Decreased sternothyroid distance

NB Predictors of difficult Trachlight (Laerdal Medical Corp, Wappingers Falls, NY, USA) lighted stylet use have been removed from this box because the Trachlight is no longer commercially available.

From Law AJ, Broemling N, Cooper RM, et al. The difficult airway with recommendations for management-part 2-the anticipated difficult airway. Can J Anaesth 2013;60:1119–38; with permission.

---

difficult airway, difficult face mask ventilation, difficult laryngoscopy (DL), DTI, difficult supraglottic device use, difficult transtracheal surgical airway, failed airway, and difficult extubation of the airway.[3]

BEDSIDE TESTS

Following several publications that were inconsistent and failed to describe the details of bedside airway tests, Lewis and colleagues[52] examined the Mallampati test and thyromental distance (TMD) measurements in 213 patients using 24 different method combinations, including neutral, sniffing, and full-extension head positions, tongue in or out, sitting and supine body positions, and presence or absence of phonation.[52] Direct laryngoscopy view was then recorded according to the definition of Cormack

---

Box 3
Predictors of difficult face mask ventilation[25–29]

- High body mass index or weight
- Older age
- Male sex
- Limited mandibular protrusion
- Decreased thyromental distance
- Modified Mallampati 3 or 4
- Beard
- Lack of teeth
- History of snoring or obstructive sleep apnea
- History of neck radiation

From Law AJ, Broemling N, Cooper RM, et al. The difficult airway with recommendations for management-part 2-the anticipated difficult airway. Can J Anaesth 2013;60:1119–38; with permission.

Box 4
Predictors of difficult supraglottic device use[30-37]

- Reduced mouth opening
- Supraglottic or extraglottic pathology (eg, neck radiation, lingual tonsillar hypertrophy)
- Glottic and subglottic pathology
- Fixed cervical spine flexion deformity
- Applied cricoid pressure
- Male sex[a]
- Increased body mass index[a]
- Poor dentition[a]
- Rotation of surgical table during case[a]
- Ear, nose, and throat procedures[b]
- Admission status[b]
- Prolonged surgical duration[b]
- Airway abnormalities[b]
- Patient transport[b]

[a]Some of the listed predictors are device specific; the 4 predictors originate from a single study using the Laryngeal Mask Airway Unique.[36]
[b]The last 5 predictors refer to failure of Laryngeal Mask Airway Unique (Teleflex Incorporated, Research Triangle Park, NC 27709, USA) and Classic in pediatric surgical patients.[113]
From Law AJ, Broemling N, Cooper RM, et al. The difficult airway with recommendations for management-part 2-the anticipated difficult airway. Can J Anaesth 2013;60:1119–38; with permission.

---

and Lehane.[48] After statistical analysis using receiver operating characteristic curves and logistic regression analysis, optimum testing conditions were defined. Recommendations from this study included performing tests with patients in the sitting position, head fully extended, tongue out, with phonation, and measuring the distance

---

Box 5
Predictors of difficult cricothyroidotomy[38,39]

- Difficulty identifying the location of the cricothyroid membrane
  - Female sex
  - Age less than 8 years
  - Thick/obese neck
  - Displaced airway
  - Overlying pathology (eg, inflammation, induration, radiation, tumor)
- Difficult access to the trachea through the anterior neck
  - Thick neck/overlying pathology
  - Fixed cervical spine flexion deformity

From Law AJ, Broemling N, Cooper RM, et al. The difficult airway with recommendations for management-part 2-the anticipated difficult airway. Can J Anaesth 2013;60:1119–38; with permission.

from the inside of the mentum to the thyroid cartilage. These results helped standardize test conditions for clinical and research purposes.

The original description of the modified Mallampati test (MMP) had the head in the neutral position.[20] The proposal by Lewis and colleagues[52] to extend the head was supported by another study by Mashour and colleagues[53] who advocate craniocervical extension during MMP testing. This position decreases the MMP class, improves specificity and positive predictive values, and maintains sensitivity.[53] A study comparing the MMP test in the supine and sitting positions in regard to Cormack Lehane scores found a higher positive predictive value and true positive values in the supine position.[54]

Using objective measurements enhances the accuracy of any test. Patil and colleagues,[55] who promoted objective measurement using a 6.5-cm thyromental gauge, first described the TMD measurement. Lewis and colleagues[52] used calipers measuring TMD in millimeters. Objective measurement of the TMD using a gauge or ruler compared with fingerbreadth measurement can treble the sensitivity of this test from 16% to 48%.[56] The inaccuracy of fingerbreadth measurement for TMD testing has been reiterated in a second study.[57] Despite these findings, the use of "three knuckles"[58] or "three ordinary finger breadths," is still advocated in some guidelines.[2]

BEDSIDE TEST REFINEMENT

Modifications to bedside tests have shown improved predictive values. An example includes the ratio of height to TMD (RHTMD). Schmitt and colleagues[59] demonstrated an increase in specificity of 91% for RHTMD compared with 73% for TMD alone. A ratio of 25 was proposed as the optimal cutoff value when predicting DL. This finding has been validated by Krobbuaban and colleagues[60] who compared the RHTMD, Mallampati test, and neck movement and found that the RHTMD had the highest odds ratio in this group (6.72 [confidence interval (CI) 3.29%–13.72%], 2.96 [1.63–5.35], and 2.73 [1.14–6.51] respectively).[60]

A study of 123 obese patients requiring tracheal intubation evaluated the neck circumference to TMD (NC/TM) as a predictive test of DTI.[61] When comparing independent predictors of DTI in obese patients including the Mallampati test and the Wilson score, the NC/TM had the best predictive outcome.

A comparison of the MMP, the upper-lip-bite test (ULBT), and the RHTMD was conducted on 603 consecutive patients with one experienced anesthesiologist performing laryngoscopy and grading according to the Cormack Lehane classification. After detailed statistical analysis, it was found that the MMP was significantly lower than the ULBT and the RHTMD scores. There was no significant difference between the ULBT and the RHTMD score.[62]

SYSTEMATIC REVIEWS

Several systematic reviews of upper airway diagnostic screening tests have been published. Lee and colleagues[63] have published a protocol pending their Cochrane review on "Airway Physical Examination Tests for Detection of Difficult Airway Management in Apparently Normal Patients."

A meta-analysis and systematic review of 6 tests was performed by Shiga and colleagues.[64] This study concluded, "Currently available screening tests for difficult intubation have only poor to moderate discriminative power when used alone. Combinations of tests add some incremental diagnostic value in comparison to the value of each test alone. The clinical value of bedside screening tests for predicting difficult intubation remains limited." This review included 25 studies and 50,760 patients. These studies were heterogeneous in terms of test methodology; the review

Table 1
Reported sensitivities, specificities and positive predictive values (PPVs) of various tests for predicting difficult tracheal intubation. (C & L is Cormack and Lehane)

Reference	Sample to Which the Derived Scoring System Was Applied	Sensitivity	Specificity	PPV	Definition of Difficulty
Derivation studies[a]					
Nath[41]	Original sample	96%	82%	31%	C & L 3-4
El-Ganzouri[11]	Original sample	~75%	~75%	≤20%	C & L 3-4/4
		~10%	~99%	~70%	—
Karkouti[42]	Original sample	~87%	96%	~31%[e]	Combination of view and no. of intubation attempts
Wilson[22]	New sample	<92%	<74%	<15%	C & L 3-4
Arne[7]	New sample	<94%	<96%	37%	Intubation aid, e.g. bougie or different blade required
Validation studies[b]					
Butler[43]	Thyromental distance	62%	25%	16%	C & L 3-4
Frerk[44]	—	7-17%	99%	15-39%	C & L 3-4/4
Frerk[44], Savva[45]	—	65-91%	81-82%	8-15%	C & L 3-4 or bougie required
Butler[43], Oates[46]	Mallampati test (original)[14]	42-56%	81-84%	4-21%	C & L 3-4
El-Ganzouri[11]	—	45-60%	87-89%	5-21%	C & L 3-4/4
Yamamoto[47]	Mallampati test (modified)[20]	65-81%	66-82%	8-9%	C & L 3-4

		45–60%	87–89%	5–21%	C & L 3-4 or bougie required
Frerk[44], Savva[45]	—				
Frerk[44]	Thyromental distance plus	81%	98%	64%	C & L 3-4 or bougie required
	Mallampati test	—	—	—	—
Oates[46], Yamamoto[47]	Wilson score[22]	42–55%	86–92%	6–9%	Epiglottis only visible/C & L 3-4
Savva[45]	Sternomental distance	82%	89%	27%	C & L 3-4 or bougie required
El-Ganzouri[11]	Mouth opening	26–47%	94–95%	7–25%	C & L 3-4/4
El-Ganzouri[11]	Neck movement	10–17%	98%	8–30%	C & L 3-4/4
El-Ganzouri[11]	Jaw protrusion	17–26%	95–96%	5–21%	C & L 3-4 or bougie required
Savva[45]		29%	85%	9%	—
Yamamoto[47]	Indirect laryngoscopy	69%	98%	31%	C & L 3-4

[a] Derivation studies – features of patients measured and used to derive a test such as scoring systems.
[b] Validation studies – predefined test(s) applied to a group of surgical patients in order to assess its (their) performance.
[c] Original sample – the one from which the scoring system was derived.
[d] C & L – Cormack & Lehane scoring system for laryngoscopy[48]; grades 3 & 4 defined in the original reference as no part of the glottis visible.
[e] Assuming an incidence of difficulty of 2%.

Adapted from Yentis SM. Predicting difficult intubation–worthwhile exercise or pointless ritual? Anaesthesia 2002;57:105–9; with permission.

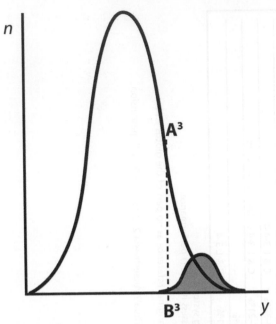

Fig. 1. A population of patients, separated into 2 overlapping groups by measuring some feature of y. In one group, tracheal intubation is easy (*clear*) and in the other it is difficult (*shaded*). The dotted line, A_3-B_3, represents the cutoff value for y.

Incidence = 5%	200 patients
Specificity ≅ 80%	10 difficult intubations
Sensitivity ≅ 90%	190 nondifficult intubations
Positive predictive value = PPV $PPV = \dfrac{9}{9+38}$ PPV=19%	9 patients identified as difficult 1 patient false negative 38 patients false positives $A_3\,B_3$ represents the cutoff value for y

(*Adapted from* Yentis SM. Predicting difficult intubation–worthwhile exercise or pointless ritual? Anesthesia 2002;57:105–9; with permission.)

was dominated by 2 studies, which accounted for 28,712 patients.[11,18] In these two studies, test methodology for TMD relied on fingerbreadth or was not defined. These two studies would, therefore, have reduced the pooled test accuracy for predicting DTI with the thyromental test.

The overall incidence of DTI in this meta-analysis was 5.8% (95% CI 4.5%–7.5%). Tests included the MMP, thyromental distance, sternomental distance, mouth opening, Wilson risk score, and a combination MMP/thyromental test. Each test showed poor to moderate sensitivity (20%–62%) and moderate to fair specificity (82%–97%).

According to the 2003 American Society of Anesthesiologists (ASA) task force on management of the difficult airway, "…there is insufficient published evidence to evaluate the effect of a physical examination in predicting the presence of a difficult airway." This report did not present a meta-analysis.[6]

The 2013 ASA task force stated, "…there is insufficient published evidence to evaluate the predictive value of multiple features of the airway physical examination versus single features in predicting the presence of a difficult airway." A meta-analysis was not presented.[2]

A meta-analysis and systematic review of the Mallampati tests[14,20] were conducted by Lee and colleagues[65] who concluded that "...the Mallampati tests have limited accuracy for predicting the difficult airway and thus are not useful screening tests."

A meta-analysis of 55 studies involving 177,088 patients examined the prognostic value of the modified Mallampati score.[50] This study concluded that "...the modified Mallampati score is inadequate as a stand-alone test of a difficult laryngoscopy or tracheal intubation, but it may well be a part of a multivariate model for the prediction of a difficult tracheal intubation."

COMPOSITE SCORING

Composite multivariable risk scores have been described to improve the predictive capability of preoperative airway assessment by combining up to 7 individual variables.[7,11,28,47,66-68] These scoring systems tend to perform better than individual variables alone; however, several deficiencies in these composite scores have been identified.[69] For example, the Wilson risk score, which tests 5 physical variables (weight, head and neck movement, jaw movement, receding mandible, and buck teeth), was designed to test DL rather than DTI.[22] Composite scores tend to be dichotomous. Langeron and colleagues[69] proposed adopting 3 classes of high, intermediate, and low risk of difficulty, as advocated by Ray and colleagues.[70] This approach creates 2 cutoff points with an intermediate, gray, or inconclusive zone. Each cutoff point can then be used to include or exclude with certainty. By developing a computer model that uses multiple simple variables, Langeron and colleagues[69] were able to accurately predict DTI and minimize the number of patients in the gray zone. This method requires further validation in various populations. It could also be used to assess other end points, such as a difficult mask ventilation or difficult supraglottic airway ventilation.[69]

THREE-COLUMN MODEL

A 3-column model of the airway has been proposed by Greenland[71,72] in an effort to provide a reliable assessment of the airway for direct laryngoscopy and tracheal intubation. This model integrates current methods of airway assessment and divides the airway into 3 columns, along with the processes of laryngoscopy and tracheal intubation. The anterior column requires evaluation of the submandibular space for laryngoscopy and includes the size of the tongue, the thyromental distance, the mandibular length, the width of the palate, and the size of the maxillary teeth. The middle column focuses on the airway passage and relies on airway history and examination, supplemented by computerized tomography and MRI scans and nasopharyngoscopy. The posterior column involves positioning of the head and neck; tests require examination of neck movement for extension and flexion. The 3-column model encourages the practitioner to inspect the airway as a whole.

RISK FACTORS

Several studies have identified risk factors associated with management of the difficult airway. Knowledge of these could help plan management and play an important role in airway assessment. Historically, examination of the airway has focused on identification of features suggestive of a DTI; but risk factors have been investigated to identify other aspects of airway difficulty, such as bag mask ventilation, laryngeal mask insertion, video laryngoscopy, and cricothyroidotomy.

Mask Ventilation

At a time of little information about the incidence or risk factors for difficult mask ventilation, Langeron and colleagues undertook a prospective study of 1502 patients, looking for these factors.[28] They defined difficult mask ventilation as "...the inability of an unassisted anesthesiologist to maintain the measured oxygen saturation as measured by pulse oximetry greater than 92%, or to prevent or reverse signs of inadequate ventilation during positive-pressure mask ventilation under general anesthesia." In this study, 75 patients had difficult mask ventilation, giving an incidence of 5% (CI 3.9%–6.1%). One patient was impossible to bag mask ventilate, and only 13 difficult mask ventilation patients were anticipated (17% of the total 75). Five independent risk factors for difficult mask ventilation were found using multivariate analysis, including age greater than 55 years, body mass index (BMI) greater than 26 kg m^{-2}, presence of a beard, lack of teeth, and a history of snoring.

Using a 4-point scale of mask ventilation difficulty, described by Han and colleagues,[73] Kheterpal and colleagues[26] prospectively studied 22,660 mask ventilation attempts. A grade 3 difficult mask ventilation incidence of 1.4% was found, and impossible mask ventilation was described in 37 patients (0.16%). Independent risk factors for difficult mask ventilation included advanced age greater than 30 years, BMI greater than 30 kg.m^{-2}, presence of a beard, and a history of snoring. Comment was also made of the association between difficult or impossible mask ventilation and DTI, whereas the mandibular protrusion test was found to be a good prognostic test; independent risk factors included a history of snoring, obstructive sleep apnea, and the presence of a thick or obese neck.

Kheterpal's study of difficult mask ventilation was not big enough to identify reliable risk factors for impossible mask ventilation.[26] A subsequent study by the same group of 53,041 mask ventilation attempts over a period of 4 years was published. Seventy-seven cases of impossible mask ventilation were found, giving an incidence of 0.15%. Independent risk factors included a history of neck radiotherapy, male sex, obstructive sleep apnea, Mallampati class III or IV, and the presence of a beard.[27] When reviewing the outcome of the 77 patients with impossible mask ventilation, only one patient required an emergency cricothyroidotomy; one was woken for an emergency tracheostomy by the surgical team; and 2 were woken for fiberoptic intubation. This finding gives a cricothyroidotomy incidence in this study of 1 patient in 53,041 or 0.0019%.

Laryngeal Mask Airways

Ramachandran and colleagues[36] have studied predictors and clinical outcomes after failed Laryngeal Mask Airway Unique (*uLMA*) (Teleflex Incorporated, Research Triangle Park, NC, USA) insertions from an adult surgical population of 15,795 patients. Failure occurred in 1.1% of the population and was associated with significant hypoxia, hypercapnia, or airway obstruction. Forty-two percent presented with inadequate ventilation related to a cuff leak. Independent risk factors for failed *uLMA* in this study were surgical table rotation, male sex, poor dentition, and increased BMI. Failed *uLMA* was also associated with a 3-fold increased incidence of difficult mask ventilation.

Video Laryngoscopes

These devices have proven high success rates for novice practitioners in patients with normal airways[74] and for experienced practitioners in patients with difficult airways.[75] Yet despite the enthusiasm for their use, they are associated with failure rates and predictors of poor clinical outcome. Experience using the GlideScope (Verathon Inc, Bothell, WA), from 2 centers, found a failure rate of 3% when used to intubate patients with anticipated difficult airways and 6% when used to rescue failed direct laryngoscopy.[23] In this study, the risk factors for GlideScope failure were altered neck anatomy, presence of a surgical scar, radiation changes, or the presence of a mass. These same risk factors apply to direct laryngoscopy. Further study is required to investigate other video laryngoscope designs, particularly in patients with difficult airways.

Difficult Mask Ventilation and Difficult Laryngoscopy

The clinical combination of difficult mask ventilation and difficult laryngoscopy is not uncommon. A recent multicenter study of 492,239 patients found 176,679 documented cases of both mask ventilation and direct laryngoscopy of which 698 were associated with difficulty. This resulted in an incidence of 0.4% of combined difficult mask ventilation and difficult laryngoscopy. From this study, 12 independent risk factors were found, including age of 46 years or older, BMI of 30 kg/m^2 or greater, male sex, Mallampati class III and IV, neck mass or radiation, limited TMD, sleep apnea, presence of teeth, presence of a beard, thick neck, limited cervical spine mobility, and limited jaw protrusion.[76]

Age

Age has also been identified as a risk factor for DTI. Moon and colleagues[77] compared young, middle-aged, and elderly adults and studied the relationship between various methods of airway assessment and the incidence and causes of DTI. The incidence of DTI was less in young adults compared with their older cohorts; the metrics associated with DTI, such as thyromental distance, cervical spine movement, interincisor distance, and grade of dentition, decreased with age, whereas the Mallampati score, cervical spine rigidity, and the ratio of Arne greater than 11 increased with age.[7,77]

Cricothyroidotomy

Cricothyroidotomy is a rare event; therefore, there are few systematic reviews of published series. A study examining the accuracy of percutaneous identification of the cricothyroid membrane in female obese and nonobese patients found that misidentification of the cricothyroid membrane was more likely in obese patients, particularly those with increased neck circumference.[38]

Neuromuscular Blocking Agents

A study conducted between 2005 and 2007 of 103,812 patients from the Danish Anesthesia Database examined whether avoiding neuromuscular blocking agents increases the risk of a DTI. In the study the incidence of DTI was 5.1% [95% confidence interval (CI): 5.0–5.3], and statistical analysis suggested that avoiding neuromuscular blocking agents increases the risk of DTI. This study also found that there was a steady decrease in the use of neuromuscular blocking agents over the period of the study, yet the frequency of DTI remained relatively unchanged. It was also found by multivariate analysis that patients who received nondepolarizing neuromuscular blocking agents were at greater risk of DTI than those who received depolarizing neuromuscular blocking agents. Other confounding factors may influence the interpretation of these results. The experience of the anesthetist and other risk factors for DTI could alter the relative importance of neuromuscular blocking agents as a risk factor for DTI.[78]

PATIENT FACTORS

In a qualitative review of 184 cases of major airway complications, identified in the Fourth National Audit Project of the Royal College of Anaesthetists and the Difficult Airway Society,[79] by an expert panel found that patient factors were the most frequent causal and contributory factors (77%) of airway complications. Certain patient factors have been found to be associated with difficult airway management and are, therefore, worth identifying in the preoperative airway assessment.

Cervical Spine Limitation

Movement of the cervical spine is an important component of direct laryngoscopy and tracheal intubation. The best position for direct laryngoscopy requires 35° neck flexion and face plane extension to 15°.[80] The Mallampati test,[53] thyromental distance,[81] and mouth opening[82] are all impaired by cervical spine limitation, which suggests the importance of adequate neck movement when trying to predict DTI. In a retrospective review of 14,053 patients, Mashour and colleagues[53] found an incidence of cervical spine limitation of 8.1%. A multivariate analysis found that cervical spine limitation was associated with increased difficulty in all aspects of airway management, and DTI could be expected in patients who had cervical spine limitation; independent risk factors included patients aged 48 years or older, TMD less than 6 cm, and Mallampati class III and IV.

Obesity

The association between obesity and DTI has been investigated in several studies, with varying conclusions concerning obesity as an independent risk factor for DTI. Some studies suggest that obesity does not increase the risk of DL[83] or DTI.[8,84] Others suggest the contrary.[11,22] A cohort study from the Danish Anesthesia Database of 91,332 consecutive patients found that obese patients with a BMI of 35 kg/m^{-2} or more did predict DTI as a stand-alone test with a sensitivity of 7.5% (95% CI 7.3%–7.7%) and a positive predictive value of 6.4% (95% CI 6.3%–6.6%).[85] The methodology and size of this study lend credibility to this result, which shows a high BMI as a weak but statistically significant predictor of difficult and failed intubation. Examining the relative impact of weight and height in this study, a univariate analysis found that these variables were statistically significant in their association with DTI; but only weight was found as an independent risk factor for DTI.

Other aspects of airway difficulty have also been related to obesity. Kheterpal and colleagues,[26] in a study of 22,660 patients, identified obesity with a BMI greater than 30 kg/m^{-2} as a risk factor for difficult mask ventilation. A study of 50 morbidly obese patients with a BMI greater than 35 kg/m^{-2} were assessed for DL using thyromental distance, mouth opening, MMP, abnormal upper teeth, neck circumference, and sleep apnea. None of these factors correlated with DL; however, patients with DL were found to have a greater neck circumference and more pretracheal soft tissue, as measured by ultrasound; these measurements correlated with difficult direct laryngoscopy.[83] Another study failed to establish increased pretracheal tissue as a predictor of DL in obese patients.[86]

Acromegaly

Acromegaly is associated with macroglossia, enlarged and distorted laryngeal anatomy, and prognathism. The incidence of DTI in patients with acromegaly is 4 to 5 times higher than people without acromegaly. In this study, only the Mallampati test had moderate predictive validity. The sensitivity and specificity to predict DL and DTI using the MMP grades 3 and 4 were 76% and 44%, respectively. The MMP test was measured with the patients in the sitting position, without phonation; the head was held in a neutral position, as described by Samsoon and Young,[20] but contrary to the optimum conditions described by Lewis and colleagues.[52] In the study group of 128 patients with acromegaly, the TMD was 9.5 ±1.5 cm (6–14 cm). This test was not predictive of DL. The difference between patients with or without DL was not significant.[87] Similar results were also found in a study by Ali and colleagues.[88]

Pregnancy

Several studies have described an increase in the Mallampati class during pregnancy and during labor.[89-91] Approximately one-third of patients were observed to increase their Mallampati score, regardless of the use of an epidural.[92] Despite these changes, a review of 2633 intubations during pregnancy found a difficult (4.7%) and failed (0.08%) intubation rate similar to the nonpregnant general surgical population. In this study, risk factors included a maternal age of 35 years or older, weight of 90 to 99 Kg, and the absence of active labor.[93]

Thyroid Hypertrophy

In 324 consecutive patients presenting for thyroid surgery, there was an overall incidence of DTI in 11.1% of patients, when assessed using the Intubating Difficulty Scale.[94] By comparison, the incidence of DTI in 1171 patients during routine surgery was 8%.[95] Palpable goiter, endothoracic goiter, thyroid malignancy, and airway deformation were not found to be specific predictors of DTI; however, MMP class 3 and 4, interdental distance less than 35 mm, TMD less than 6.5 cm, cervical spine limitation less than 80°, short neck, and retrognathia were significantly reliable predictors of DTI.[96]

HISTORY OF A PREVIOUS DIFFICULT TRACHEAL INTUBATION

A study of 103,812 patients from the Danish Anesthesia Database assessed the diagnostic accuracy of a previous documented DTI. It was found that 24% (21%–28%) of patients who had previously experienced difficulty with direct laryngoscopy and tracheal intubation also experienced difficulty with tracheal intubation on another occasion. Conversely, of the patients who experienced no difficulty with tracheal intubation, 95% (95%–95%) had the same outcome during a subsequent event. A repeat experience of a failed direct laryngoscopy and tracheal intubation occurred 30% (24%–36%) of the time, compared with the patients who did not experience a failed intubation, whereas 98% (98%–98%) did not experience a subsequent failed tracheal intubation by direct laryngoscopy. Using a multivariate regression model and adjusting for other covariates, an odds ratio of 16.6 (11.9–23.2, 95% CI, $P<.0001$) suggested that a previous failed tracheal intubation by direct laryngoscopy was a strong predictor for future failed intubation.[97]

OTHER TESTS

Various forms of imaging, indirect visualization, and mathematical modeling have been proposed to predict the difficult airway.

Nasopharyngoscopy

Indirect visualization of the upper airway by nasopharyngoscopy is a quick and potentially rewarding clinical examination of patients who have known or suspected upper airway pathology. Information derived from this examination can direct airway management. In a prospective study of 140 patients presenting for diagnostic or therapeutic airway procedures by Rosenblatt and colleagues,[98] a preoperative endoscopic airway examination (PEAE) was performed following a standard airway examination and management plan. In 26% of patients, the PEAE had an influence on the original airway management plan.

Ultrasound

Ultrasonography has a limited role in predicting DTI when interpretation of the scan can be difficult.[99,100] The floor of the mouth can be seen, but the epiglottis is problematic because it is surrounded by air.[101] Despite these limitations, ultrasonography can be useful evaluating the airway for subglottic tumors, assessing fasting status, and diagnosing obstructive sleep apnea.[102] Identification of the cricothyroid membrane with ultrasonography can be achieved with a mean time of 24.3 seconds, which is a useful aid considering percutaneous identification of anatomic landmarks has a success rate of only 30%.[39,103] Preoperative identification of the trachea in adults and children is also possible with ultrasonography, where percutaneous palpation or radiology can fail.[104,105] Studies have used ultrasound to measure the hyomental ratio, base of tongue mass, and pretracheal distance; but there is inadequate evidence to support these measurements as screening tests to identify difficult airways.[106]

Computer Analysis

A computer software analysis of facial photographs created a computer model that could objectively analyze facial anatomy to improve the prediction of a difficult intubation. This analysis, which included 3 facial parameters, was combined with the thyromental test and used to analyze 80 male subjects who had been divided into easy and challenging intubation groups. The technique correctly classified 70 of 80 subjects, compared with an MMP/TMD test combination, which correctly classified 47 of 80. Sensitivity, specificity, and area under the curve for the computer modeling method were 90%, 85%, and 0.899, respectively. This study measured TMD with fingerbreadths and with the patients' head in the neutral position, both of which are known to significantly decrease this test's sensitivity compared with objective measurement of the TMD,[56] and head extension.[52]

LIMITATIONS OF AIRWAY TESTS IN EMERGENCY MEDICINE, INTENSIVE CARE, AND PEDIATRICS

Various limitations of predictive tests used in airway assessment have been identified. Patients in the emergency department, who require tracheal intubation, may be obtunded or uncooperative, rendering predictive tests inappropriate. Levitan and colleagues[107] found that all of the rapid sequence intubation failures and two-thirds of the non–cardiac arrest emergency medicine intubations were inappropriate for predictive tests, such as the Mallampati score, TMD, and neck mobility measurement. These findings were reinforced by Bair and colleagues[108] who questioned the feasibility of a preoperative Mallampati test in the emergency department after studying 296 adult emergency patients requiring tracheal intubation. They found only 76 patients (26%) (CI 21%–31%) were able to comply with a Mallampati test, citing lack of patient cooperation and clinical instability as reasons for this low result.

DTI in the intensive care unit (ICU) is associated with high mortality.[109] An intubation score has been developed and independently validated in a multicenter trial. The score is based on patient, pathology, and operator factors. Called the MACOCHA score, factors and weighted scores include Mallampati class III and IV (5 points), apnea syndrome (obstructive) (2 points), cervical spine limitation (1 point), opening mouth less than 3 cm (1 point), coma (1 point), hypoxia (1 point), and anesthesiologist nontrained (1 point). The 12-point score has limits of zero (easy) and 12 (very difficult). The score was prospectively developed from 1000 consecutive intubations in a multicenter study, including 42 ICUs, and then validated with 400 consecutive intubations from a separate 18 ICUs. In the validation study, the MACOCHA score sensitivity was 73%, specificity 89%, negative predictive value 98%, and positive predictive value 36%. Thirty-eight percent of the 1000 cases experienced severe life-threatening events, including severe hypoxia, collapse, cardiac arrest, or death. Using the MACOCHA score, a significantly higher incidence of life-threatening complications was found in the difficult intubation group compared with the nondifficult intubation group (51% vs 36%, P .0001).[110]

Airway assessment in the context of retrieval medicine has not yet been described; however, management in these environments is likely to involve the same challenges as those described in emergency medicine and intensive care.

Pediatric patients, whose ages range from birth to 16 years, present with a broad spectrum of anatomic features, which is incompatible with tests using fixed end points, such as the TMD. Young children are often uncooperative or unable to comply with simple instructions when performing airway tests. A study of 476 infants and children examined the predictive capability of the Mallampati test for DTI. Five pediatric anesthetists recorded a Samsoon and Young modified Mallampati test, using a tongue blade to open the mouth if necessary. They then performed direct laryngoscopy with a laryngoscope of their choice. The Mallampati test was found to have overall sensitivity of 16.2% with 9.6% in children less than 3 years of age and 22.0% in children older than 3 years. The specificity and positive predictive values were not reported. This study can be criticized for nonstandard application of the Mallampati test, use of a variety of laryngoscopes to achieve a laryngeal view as described by the Cormack Lehane scale, and failure to rate intubation difficulty. The sensitivity was unacceptably low indicating that the Mallampati test is inaccurate and is not a useful screening test in this age group.[111]

A second pediatric study found that the Mallampati test was applicable in children aged 4 to 8 years when correlated with the Cormack Lehane scale for direct laryngoscopy. This study found a sensitivity of 75.8% (CI 21.9%–98.7%) and specificity of 96.2% (CI 89.9%–98.9%).[112] The wide CIs for sensitivity suggest that the Mallampati test may include many false-positive cases. The lack of reliability of the Mallampati test to correctly predict DTI in this study is demonstrated by the positive predictive value of 42.9% (CI 11.8%–79.8%).

A retrospective data base review of 11,910 pediatric patients anaesthetized with a laryngeal mask airway (LMA) found a failure rate of 0.86%. This finding compared favorably with a similar adult study that reported a failure rate of 1.1%.[36] Presenting features in the pediatric study included LMA leak, obstruction, and patient intolerance. Independent risk factors associated with failure included ear nose and throat surgery, nonoutpatient admission status, prolonged surgical duration, congenital/acquired airway abnormality, and patient transport.[113]

In a retrospective analysis of 11,219 pediatric anesthesia patients up to 18 years of age, it was found that the incidence of DL (as defined by Cormack Lehane grade III and IV) is lower in children (1.35%)[114] than in adults (9.0%).[40] Infants had a higher incidence of DL than older patients (4.7% vs 0.7%). Risk factors in this study included children undergoing cardiac and oromaxillofacial surgery, ASA physical status II and IV, Mallampati class III and IV, and children with a low BMI.

A review of pediatric syndromes and medical conditions identified anatomic predictors of pediatric DTI, including reduced head extension, reduced mandibular space, and increased anteroposterior tongue thickness.[115]

SUMMARY

Assessment of the airway is an important component of preparing patients for safe airway management. Improving the prediction of difficult airways can be achieved by adopting objective assessment. Review of the literature suggests that bedside airway tests are very poor predictors of airway difficulty. Improvements can be achieved, however, by adopting combined tests or by using indices, such as the ratio of height to TMD. Knowledge of risk factors associated with particular clinical conditions may also assist in the planning of safe airway management. There are still important gaps in our knowledge of optimizing assessment of the airway, but the important consequence of airway assessment is the development of an airway management plan.

REFERENCES

1. The good anaesthetist. Standards of practice for career grade anaesthetists. London: The Royal College of Anaesthetists; 2010. Available at: http://www. rcoa.ac.uk/document-store/the-good-anaesthetist. Accessed May 11, 2014.
2. Practice Guidelines for Management of the Difficult Airway. An Updated Report by the American Society of Anesthesiologists Task Force on Management of the Difficult Airway. Anesthesiology 2013;118:251–70.
3. Law AJ, Broemling N, Cooper RM, et al. The difficult airway with recommendations for management-Part 1-Difficult tracheal intubation encountered in an unconscious/induced patient. Can J Anaesth 2013;60.
4. Law AJ, Broemling N, Cooper RM, et al. The difficult airway with recommendations for management-Part 2-The anticipated difficult airway. Can J Anaesth 2013;60:1119–38.
5. Cass NM, James NR, Lines V. Difficult direct laryngoscopy complicating intubation for anaesthesia. Br Med J 1956;1:488–9.
6. Practise Guidelines for Management of the Difficult Airway. An Updated Report by the American Society of Anesthesiologists Task Force on Management of the Difficult Airway. Anesthesiology 2003;98:1269–77.
7. Arne J, Descoins P, Fusciardi J, et al. Preoperative assessment for difficult intubation in general and ENT surgery: predictive value of a clinical multivariate risk index. Br J Anaesth 1998;80:140–6.
8. Brodsky JB, Lemmens HJ, Brock-Utne JG, et al. Morbid obesity and tracheal intubation. Anesth Analg 2002;94:732–6. Table of contents.
9. Eberhart LH, Arndt C, Aust HJ, et al. A simplified risk score to predict difficult intubation: development and prospective evaluation in 3763 patients. Eur J Anaesthesiol 2010;27:935–40.
10. Eberhart LH, Arndt C, Cierpka T, et al. The reliability and validity of the upper lip bite test compared with the Mallampati classification to predict difficult laryngoscopy: an external prospective evaluation. Anesth Analg 2005;101:284–9. Table of contents.
11. el-Ganzouri AR, McCarthy RJ, Tuman KJ, et al. Preoperative airway assessment: predictive value of a multivariate risk index. Anesth Analg 1996;82:1197–204.
12. Karkouti K, Rose DK, Ferris LE, et al. Inter-observer reliability of ten tests used for predicting difficult tracheal intubation. Can J Anaesth 1996;43:554–9.

13. Khan ZH, Gharabaghian M, Nilli F, et al. Easy endotracheal intubation of a patient suffering from both Cushing's and Nelson's syndromes predicted by the upper lip bite test despite a Mallampati Class 4 airway. Anesth Analg 2007;105:786–7.
14. Mallampati SR, Gatt SP, Gugino LD, et al. A clinical sign to predict difficult tracheal intubation: a prospective study. Can Anaesth Soc J 1985;32:429–34.
15. Orozco-Diaz E, Alvarez-Rios JJ, Arceo-Diaz JL, et al. Predictive factors of difficult airway with known assessment scales. Cir Cir 2010;78:393–9.
16. Reed MJ, Dunn MJ, McKeown DW. Can an airway assessment score predict intubation success in the emergency department? Emerg Med Australas 2005;17: 94–6.
17. Rocke DA, Murray WB, Rout CC, et al. Relative risk analysis of factors associated with difficult intubation in obstetric anesthesia. Anesthesiology 1992;77:67–73.
18. Rose DK, Cohen MM. The airway: problems and predictions in 18,500 patients. Can J Anaesth 1994;41:372–83.
19. Saghaei M, Safavi MR. Prediction of prolonged laryngoscopy. Anaesthesia 2001; 56:1198–201.
20. Samsoon GL, Young JR. Difficult tracheal intubation: a retrospective study. Anaesthesia 1987;42:487–90.
21. Tse JC, Rimm EB, Hussain A. Predicting difficult endotracheal intubation in surgical patients scheduled for general anesthesia: a prospective blind study. Anesth Analg 1995;81:254–8.
22. Wilson ME, Spiegelhalter D, Robertson JA, et al. Predicting difficult intubation. Br J Anaesth 1988;61:211–6.
23. Aziz MF, Healy D, Kheterpal S, et al. Routine clinical practice effectiveness of the Glidescope in difficult airway management: an analysis of 2,004 Glidescope intubations, complications, and failures from two institutions. Anesthesiology 2011;114:34–41.
24. Tremblay MH, Williams S, Robitaille A, et al. Poor visualization during direct laryngoscopy and high upper lip bite test score are predictors of difficult intubation with the GlideScope videolaryngoscope. Anesth Analg 2008;106:1495–500. Table of contents.
25. Gautam P, Gaul TK, Luthra N. Prediction of difficult mask ventilation. Eur J Anaesthesiol 2005;22:638–40.
26. Kheterpal S, Han R, Tremper KK, et al. Incidence and predictors of difficult and impossible mask ventilation. Anesthesiology 2006;105:885–91.
27. Kheterpal S, Martin L, Shanks AM, et al. Prediction and outcomes of impossible mask ventilation: a review of 50,000 anesthetics. Anesthesiology 2009;110: 891–7.
28. Langeron O, Masso E, Huraux C, et al. Prediction of difficult mask ventilation. Anesthesiology 2000;92:1229–36.
29. Yildiz TS, Solak M, Toker K. The incidence and risk factors of difficult mask ventilation. J Anesth 2005;19:7–11.
30. Asai T, Hirose T, Shingu K. Failed tracheal intubation using a laryngoscope and intubating laryngeal mask. Can J Anaesth 2000;47:325–8.
31. Giraud O, Bourgain JL, Marandas P, et al. Limits of laryngeal mask airway in patients after cervical or oral radiotherapy. Can J Anaesth 1997;44:1237–41.
32. Ishimura H, Minami K, Sata T, et al. Impossible insertion of the laryngeal mask airway and oropharyngeal axes. Anesthesiology 1995;83:867–9.
33. Kumar R, Prashast, Wadhwa A, et al. The upside-down intubating laryngeal mask airway: a technique for cases of fixed flexed neck deformity. Anesth Analg 2002; 95:1454–8. Table of contents.

34. Langeron O, Semjen F, Bourgain JL, et al. Comparison of the intubating laryngeal mask airway with the fiberoptic intubation in anticipated difficult airway management. Anesthesiology 2001;94:968–72.
35. Li CW, Xue FS, Xu YC, et al. Cricoid pressure impedes insertion of, and ventilation through, the ProSeal laryngeal mask airway in anesthetized, paralyzed patients. Anesth Analg 2007;104:1195–8. Tables of contents.
36. Ramachandran SK, Mathis MR, Tremper KK, et al. Predictors and clinical outcomes from failed Laryngeal Mask Airway UniqueTM: a study of 15,795 patients. Anesthesiology 2012;116:1217–26.
37. Salvi L, Juliano G, Zucchetti M, et al. Hypertrophy of the lingual tonsil and difficulty in airway control. A clinical case. Minerva Anestesiol 1999;65:549–53.
38. Aslani A, Ng SC, Hurley M, et al. Accuracy of identification of the cricothyroid membrane in female subjects using palpation: an observational study. Anesth Analg 2012;114:987–92.
39. Elliott DS, Baker PA, Scott MR, et al. Accuracy of surface landmark identification for cannula cricothyroidotomy. Anaesthesia 2010;65:889–94 [Erratum appears in Anaesthesia 2010;65(12):1258].
40. Yentis SM. Predicting difficult intubation–worthwhile exercise or pointless ritual? Anaesthesia 2002;57:105–9.
41. Nath G, Sekar M. Predicting difficult intubation–a comprehensive scoring system. Anaesth Intensive Care 1997;25:482–6.
42. Karkouti K, Rose DK, Ferris LE, et al. Inter-observer reliability of ten tests used for predicting difficult tracheal intubation [see comment]. Can J Anaesth 1996;43:554–9.
43. Butler PJ, Dhara SS. Prediction of difficult laryngoscopy: an assessment of the thyromental distance and Mallampati predictive tests [see comment]. Anaesth Intensive Care 1992;20:139–42.
44. Frerk CM. Predicting difficult intubation. Anaesthesia 1991;46:1005–8.
45. Savva D. Prediction of difficult tracheal intubation [see comment]. Br J Anaesth 1994;73:149–53.
46. Oates JD, Macleod AD, Oates PD, et al. Comparison of two methods for predicting difficult intubation. Br J Anaesth 1991;66:305–9.
47. Yamamoto K, Tsubokawa T, Shibata K, et al. Predicting difficult intubation with indirect laryngoscopy. Anesthesiology 1997;86:316–21.
48. Cormack RS, Lehane J. Difficult tracheal intubation in obstetrics. Anaesthesia 1984;39:1105–11.
49. Adamus M, Jor O, Vavreckova T, et al. Inter-observer reproducibility of 15 tests used for predicting difficult intubation. Biomed Pap Med Fac Univ Palacky Olomouc Czech Repub 2011;155:275–81.
50. Lundstrom LH, Vester-Andersen M, Moller AM, et al, Danish Anaesthesia Database. Poor prognostic value of the modified Mallampati score: a meta-analysis involving 177 088 patients. Br J Anaesth 2011;107:659–67.
51. Frova G, Sorbello M. Algorithms for difficult airway management: a review. Minerva Anestesiol 2009;75:201–9.
52. Lewis MM, Keramati SM, Benumof JL, et al. What is the best way to determine oropharyngeal classification and mandibular space length to predict difficult laryngoscopy? Anesthesiology 1994;81:69–75.
53. Mashour GA, Stallmer ML, Kheterpal S, et al. Predictors of difficult intubation in patients with cervical spine limitations. J Neurosurg Anesthesiol 2008;20:110–5.
54. Bindra A, Prabhakar H, Singh GP, et al. Is the modified Mallampati test performed in supine position a reliable predictor of difficult tracheal intubation? J Anesth 2010;24:482–5 [Erratum appears in J Anesth 2011;25(1):137].

55. Patil VS, Zauder HL. Predicting the difficulty of intubation utilizing an intubation gauge. Anesthesiol Rev 1983;X:32–3.
56. Baker PA, Depuydt A, Thompson JM. Thyromental distance measurement–fingers don't rule. Anaesthesia 2009;64:878–82.
57. Kiser M, Wakim JA, Hill L. Accuracy of fingerbreadth measurements for thyromental distance estimates: a brief report. AANA J 2011;79:15–8.
58. Seo SH, Lee JG, Yu SB, et al. Predictors of difficult intubation defined by the intubation difficulty scale (IDS): predictive value of 7 airway assessment factors. Korean J Anesthesiol 2012;63:491–7.
59. Schmitt HJ, Kirmse M, Radespiel-Troger M. Ratio of patient's height to thyromental distance improves prediction of difficult laryngoscopy. Anaesth Intensive Care 2002;30:763–5.
60. Krobbuaban B, Diregpoke S, Kumkeaw S, et al. The predictive value of the height ratio and thyromental distance: four predictive tests for difficult laryngoscopy. Anesth Analg 2005;101:1542–5.
61. Kim WH, Ahn HJ, Lee CJ, et al. Neck circumference to thyromental distance ratio: a new predictor of difficult intubation in obese patients. Br J Anaesth 2011;106:743–8.
62. Safavi M, Honarmand A, Zare N. A comparison of the ratio of patient's height to thyromental distance with the modified Mallampati and the upper lip bite test in predicting difficult laryngoscopy. Saudi J Anaesth 2011;5:258–63.
63. Lee A, Herkner H, Hovhannisyan K, et al. Airway physical examination tests for detection of difficult airway management in apparently normal patients. Cochrane Database Syst Rev 2012;(5). 00075320–100000000-07269.
64. Shiga T, Wajima Z, Inoue T, et al. Predicting difficult intubation in apparently normal patients: a meta-analysis of bedside screening test performance. Anesthesiology 2005;103:429–37.
65. Lee A, Fan LT, Gin T, et al. A systematic review (meta-analysis) of the accuracy of the Mallampati tests to predict the difficult airway. Anesth Analg 2006;102:1867–78.
66. L'Hermite J, Nouvellon E, Cuvillon P, et al. The Simplified Predictive Intubation Difficulty Score: a new weighted score for difficult airway assessment. Eur J Anaesthesiol 2009;26:1003–9.
67. Naguib M, Scamman FL, O'Sullivan C, et al. Predictive performance of three multivariate difficult tracheal intubation models: a double-blind, case-controlled study. Anesth Analg 2006;102:818–24.
68. Wilson ME. Predicting difficult intubation. Br J Anaesth 1993;71:333–4.
69. Langeron O, Cuvillon P, Ibanez-Esteve C, et al. Prediction of difficult tracheal intubation: time for a paradigm change. Anesthesiology 2012;117:1223–33.
70. Ray PM, Manach YL, Riou BM, et al. Statistical Evaluation of a Biomarker. Anesthesiology 2010;112:1023–40.
71. Greenland KB. A proposed model for direct laryngoscopy and tracheal intubation. Anaesthesia 2008;63:156–61.
72. Greenland KB. Airway assessment based on a three column model of direct laryngoscopy. Anaesth Intensive Care 2010;38:14–9.
73. Han R, Tremper KK, Kheterpal S, et al. Grading scale for mask ventilation. Anesthesiology 2004;101:267.
74. Nouruzi-Sedeh P, Schumann M, Groeben H. Laryngoscopy via Macintosh blade versus GlideScope: success rate and time for endotracheal intubation in untrained medical personnel. Anesthesiology 2009;110:32–7.
75. Aziz MF, Dillman D, Fu R, et al. Comparative effectiveness of the C-MAC video laryngoscope versus direct laryngoscopy in the setting of the predicted difficult airway. Anesthesiology 2012;116:629–36.

76. Kheterpal S, Healy D, Aziz MF, et al. Incidence, predictors, and outcome of difficult mask ventilation combined with difficult laryngoscopy. Anesthesiology 2013; 119:1360–9.

77. Moon HY, Baek CW, Kim JS, et al. The causes of difficult tracheal intubation and preoperative assessments in different age groups. Korean J Anesthesiol 2013;64: 308–14.

78. Lundstrom LH, Moller AM, Rosenstock C, et al, Danish Anaesthesia Database. Avoidance of neuromuscular blocking agents may increase the risk of difficult tracheal intubation: a cohort study of 103,812 consecutive adult patients recorded in the Danish Anaesthesia Database. Br J Anaesth 2009;103:283–90.

79. Cook TM, Woodall N, Frerk C. Major complications of airway management in the UK: results of the Fourth National Audit Project of the Royal College of Anaesthetists and the Difficult Airway Society. Part 1: anaesthesia. Br J Anaesth 2011;106:617–31.

80. Greenland KB, Edwards MJ, Hutton NJ, et al. Changes in airway configuration with different head and neck positions using magnetic resonance imaging of normal airways: a new concept with possible clinical applications. Br J Anaesth 2010;105:683–90.

81. Qudaisat IY, Al-Ghanem SM. Short thyromental distance is a surrogate for inadequate head extension, rather than small submandibular space, when indicating possible difficult direct laryngoscopy. Eur J Anaesthesiol 2011;28:600–6.

82. Calder I, Picard J, Chapman M, et al. Mouth opening: a new angle. Anesthesiology 2003;99:799–801.

83. Ezri T, Gewurtz G, Sessler DI, et al. Prediction of difficult laryngoscopy in obese patients by ultrasound quantification of anterior neck soft tissue. Anaesthesia 2003;58:1111–4.

84. Bond A. Obesity and difficult intubation. Anaesth Intensive Care 1993;21:828–30.

85. Lundstrom LH, Moller AM, Rosenstock C, et al. High body mass index is a weak predictor for difficult and failed tracheal intubation: a cohort study of 91,332 consecutive patients scheduled for direct laryngoscopy registered in the Danish Anesthesia Database. Anesthesiology 2009;110:266–74.

86. Komatsu R, Sengupta P, Wadhwa A, et al. Ultrasound quantification of anterior soft tissue thickness fails to predict difficult laryngoscopy in obese patients. Anaesth Intensive Care 2007;35:32–7.

87. Schmitt H, Buchfelder M, Radespiel-Troger M, et al. Difficult intubation in acromegalic patients: incidence and predictability. Anesthesiology 2000;93:110–4.

88. Ali Z, Bithal PK, Prabhakar H, et al. An assessment of the predictors of difficult intubation in patients with acromegaly. J Clin Neurosci 2009;16:1043–5.

89. Boutonnet M, Faitot V, Katz A, et al. Mallampati class changes during pregnancy, labour, and after delivery: can these be predicted? Br J Anaesth 2010;104:67–70.

90. Kodali BS, Chandrasekhar S, Bulich LN, et al. Airway changes during labor and delivery. Anesthesiology 2008;108:357–62.

91. Pilkington S, Carli F, Dakin MJ, et al. Increase in Mallampati score during pregnancy. Br J Anaesth 1995;74:638–42.

92. Guru R, Carere MD, Diwan S, et al. Effect of epidural analgesia on change in Mallampati class during labour. Anaesthesia 2013;68:765–9.

93. McKeen DM, George RB, O'Connell CM, et al. Difficult and failed intubation: Incident rates and maternal, obstetrical, and anesthetic predictors. Can J Anaesth 2011;58:514–24.

94. Adnet F, Borron SW, Racine SX, et al. The intubation difficulty scale (IDS): proposal and evaluation of a new score characterizing the complexity of endotracheal intubation. Anesthesiology 1997;87:1290–7.

95. Adnet F, Racine SX, Borron SW, et al. A survey of tracheal intubation difficulty in the operating room: a prospective observational study. Acta Anaesthesiol Scand 2001;45:327–32.

96. Amathieu R, Smail N, Catineau J, et al. Difficult intubation in thyroid surgery: myth or reality? Anesth Analg 2006;103:965–8.

97. Lundstrom LH, Moller AM, Rosenstock C, et al, Danish Anaesthesia Database. A documented previous difficult tracheal intubation as a prognostic test for a subsequent difficult tracheal intubation in adults. Anaesthesia 2009;64:1081–8.

98. Rosenblatt W, Ianus AI, Sukhupragarn W, et al. Preoperative endoscopic airway examination (PEAE) provides superior airway information and may reduce the use of unnecessary awake intubation. Anesth Analg 2011;112:602–7.

99. Tsui BC, Hui CM. Sublingual airway ultrasound imaging. Can J Anaesth 2008;55:790–1.

100. Tsui BC, Hui CM. Challenges in sublingual airway ultrasound interpretation. Can J Anaesth 2009;56:393–4.

101. Kundra P, Mishra SK, Ramesh A. Ultrasound of the airway. Indian J Anaesth 2011;55:456–62.

102. Kristensen MS. Ultrasonography in the management of the airway. Acta Anaesthesiol Scand 2011;55:1155–73.

103. Nicholls SE, Sweeney TW, Ferre RM, et al. Bedside sonography by emergency physicians for the rapid identification of landmarks relevant to cricothyrotomy. Am J Emerg Med 2008;26:852–6.

104. Emshoff R, Bertram S, Kreczy A. Topographic variations in anatomical structures of the anterior neck of children: an ultrasonographic study. Oral Surg Oral Med Oral Pathol Oral Radiol Endod 1999;87:429–36.

105. Munir N, Hughes D, Sadera G, et al. Ultrasound-guided localisation of trachea for surgical tracheostomy. Eur Arch Otorhinolaryngol 2010;267:477–9.

106. Kristensen MS, Teoh WH, Graumann O, et al. Ultrasonography for clinical decision-making and intervention in airway management: from the mouth to the lungs and pleurae. Insights Imaging 2014;5:253–79.

107. Levitan RM, Everett WW, Ochroch EA. Limitations of difficult airway prediction in patients intubated in the emergency department. Ann Emerg Med 2004;44:307–13.

108. Bair AE, Caravelli R, Tyler K, et al. Feasibility of the preoperative Mallampati airway assessment in emergency department patients. J Emerg Med 2010;38:677–80.

109. Jaber S, Amraoui J, Lefrant JY, et al. Clinical practice and risk factors for immediate complications of endotracheal intubation in the intensive care unit: a prospective, multiple-center study. Crit Care Med 2006;34:2355–61.

110. De Jong A, Molinari N, Terzi N, et al, AzuRea Network for the Frida-Rea Study Group. Early identification of patients at risk for difficult intubation in the intensive care unit: development and validation of the MACOCHA score in a multicenter cohort study. Am J Respir Crit Care Med 2013;187:832–9.

111. Koop VJ, Baily A, Valley RD, et al. Utility of the Mallampati classification for predicting difficult intubation in pediatric patients. Anesthesiology 1995;83:A1147.

112. Santos AP, Mathias LA, Gozzani JL, et al. Difficult intubation in children: applicability of the Mallampati index. Rev Bras Anestesiol 2011;61:156–8, 159–62, 84–7.

113. Mathis MR, Haydar B, Taylor EL, et al. Failure of the Laryngeal Mask Airway and Classic in the Pediatric Surgical Patient. Anesthesiology 2013;119:1284–95.

114. Heinrich S, Birkholz T, Ihmsen H, et al. Incidence and predictors of difficult laryngoscopy in 11,219 pediatric anesthesia procedures. Paediatr Anaesth 2012;22: 729–36.

115. Frei FJ, Ummenhofer W. Difficult intubation in paediatrics. Paediatr Anaesth 1996;6:251–63.

Predictors of Difficult Intubation and the Otolaryngology Perioperative Consult

Karla O'Dell, MD

KEYWORDS

- Difficult intubation • Airway management • Airway obstruction

KEY POINTS

- It is critical to identify patients with a difficult airway to mobilize sufficient physician and support staff, to ensure that airway management equipment is available, and to prepare the patient.
- History of prior difficult intubation, head and neck radiation, congenital malformations, cervical spine disease, obesity, and obstructive sleep apnea can be associated with increased difficulty in intubation.
- Physical examination findings of decreased mouth opening, Mallampati score, decreased neck extension, and increased neck circumference are associated with difficulty in intubation.
- When selecting an airway management plan, it is important to decide on an approach that successfully addresses the anatomic reason for the predicted difficulty with the tracheal intubation.
- Successful management of complex airway problems is a coordinated effort between multiple specialties and nursing support staff.

INTRODUCTION

The incidence of difficulties related to airway intubation is low (1%–5.8%),[1-3] but failure to secure an airway can have serious consequences, including death, brain injury, and cardiopulmonary arrest.[4] Mistakes in the algorithm for difficult intubation are mainly caused by unpreparedness.[5] Recognition of those patients for whom intubation is expected to be difficult is critical to avoid morbidity and mortality associated with a difficult intubation. Early recognition of a complex airway allows for consultation services to assist and ensures that proper equipment is readily

Department of Otolaryngology, Head and Neck Surgery, Keck School of Medicine, University of Southern California, 1450 San Pablo Street, Los Angeles, CA 90033, USA
E-mail address: kodell@usc.edu

Anesthesiology Clin 33 (2015) 279–290
http://dx.doi.org/10.1016/j.anclin.2015.02.002
1932-2275/15/$ – see front matter © 2015 Elsevier Inc. All rights reserved.

available and all staff are prepared. An airway history and physical examination should be conducted, when feasible, before the initiation of anesthetic care and airway management in all patients.[4] The purpose of the airway evaluation is to detect medical, physical, and surgical factors that may indicate the presence of a difficult airway. There are certain predictors of anticipated difficulty with intubation, but no individual factor or prediction model offers 100% sensitivity.[3,6,7] Therefore, multiple history and examination findings should be used to help predict difficult intubation. When a difficult intubation is anticipated, otolaryngologists and anesthesiologists should jointly plan the management of the difficult airway to ensure successful control.

DEFINITION OF A DIFFICULT AIRWAY

There is no standard accepted definition of a difficult airway. The anesthesiology practice management guidelines define a difficult airway as a clinical situation in which a trained anesthesiologist experiences difficulty with face mask ventilation of the upper airway, difficulty with tracheal intubation, or both.[4,8]

- Difficult mask ventilation is when it is not possible to provide adequate mask ventilation because of inadequate mask seal, excessive gas leak, or excessive resistance. Signs of inadequate face mask ventilation include absent or minimal chest rise, absent or inadequate breath sounds, ausculatory signs of obstruction, cyanosis, decreasing or inadequate oxygen saturation, absent or inadequate spirometric measures of exhaled gas flow, absent or inadequate exhaled carbon dioxide, and hemodynamic changes associated with hypoxemia.[4,8]
- Difficult laryngoscopy is when it is not possible to visualize any portion of the vocal folds after multiple attempts at conventional laryngoscopy with external compression. This condition is also known as a Cormack-Lehane laryngeal grade 3 or 4 views (**Box 1**).[9]
- Difficult tracheal intubation is tracheal intubation that requires multiple attempts in the presence or absence of tracheal disorder.
- Failed intubation occurs when placement of endotracheal tube fails after multiple attempts.

EVALUATION

An airway evaluation should be performed on every patient requiring airway management.[5] This evaluation should include key information in the patient's history and physical examination that may affect endotracheal tube placement. There

---

Box 1
Cormack-Lehane scale

Grade 1: full view of glottis

Grade 2: partial vocal fold/posterior commissure

Grade 3: epiglottic tip visualized

Grade 4: no exposure of glottic structures

From Cormack RS, Lehane J. Difficult tracheal intubation in obstetrics. Anesthesia 1984;39(11):1106.

should be an assessment of not only the predicted ease or difficulty of tracheal intubation but also the predicted success of fallback options to achieve oxygenation, such as face mask ventilation, laryngeal mask airway (LMA), and surgical airway.

History

Previous history of difficult intubation

A history of a prior difficult intubation or failed intubation can be an indication of difficulties with future intubations (**Box 2**).[10] Lundstrom and colleagues[2] found that 24% of the patients with a documented history of difficult prior intubation subsequently experienced a difficult tracheal intubation. Among the patients with no history of difficult intubation, 95% of them subsequently underwent an intubation with no difficulty. If possible, previous anesthesia records should be reviewed to determine the factors that specifically contributed to the difficult intubation. It is challenging to rely solely on a patient's interpretation of the situation. When a difficult intubation is encountered it is also important to document the primary difficulties encountered and detail the successful and unsuccessful airway management techniques.[11]

Head and neck radiation

A history of prior head and neck radiation can contribute to difficulties with intubation. Radiation therapy results in fibrosis of tissue in the treated areas and loss of lymphatic drainage, which can cause lymphedema.[12] Fibrosis and loss of tissue pliability can cause trismus, restricted mouth opening, and a significant decrease in neck extension. Glottic and epiglottic edema secondary to radiation impedes the visualization of the glottis aperture during laryngoscopy. Fibrosis can cause significant distortion of laryngeal anatomy. Iseli and colleagues[13] showed that previous head and neck radiation was associated with failure of the first intubation plan. The use of a video laryngoscope or GlideScope can overcome some of the specific challenges to intubating a patient with prior head and neck radiation.[14] If a patient has a history of prior head and neck radiation, preoperative evaluation of the airway or consultation with the treating otolaryngologist should be considered.

Obstructive sleep apnea

There are several anatomic characteristics associated with obstructive sleep apnea (OSA), including retrognathia, increased neck circumference, and a large tongue.[15–17] These similar anatomic features make direct laryngoscopy and intubation more difficult.[18] It is therefore expected that patients with a history of sleep apnea may also be difficult to intubate. Kurtipek and colleagues[16] found significant

---

Box 2
Medical history predictors of difficult intubation

Obstructive sleep apnea Apnea-Hypopnea Index greater than 40[15,20]

Prior difficult intubation[2]

Obesity[17,21,22]

Cervical spine disease[27]

Head and neck radiation[12,13]

Congenital malformations[32,33]

differences between OSA and non-OSA groups in terms of body mass index, Mallampati grading, laryngoscopic grading, and an increase in difficult intubation. It is important to review the sleep study, focusing on the apnea-hypopnea index (AHI). The AHI measure the average number of apneas or hypopneas per hour, with 5 to 14 indicating mild sleep apnea, 15 to 30 indicating moderate, and greater than 30 indicating severe.[19] Patients with an AHI of greater than 40 (severe sleep apnea) have a significantly higher risk of a difficult intubation.[15,17,20] Kim and Lee[20] showed that patients with severe OSA had a 16% incidence compared with 3.3% in the control (non-OSA) group.

Obesity

Obesity can also be a factor that may contribute to difficulties with mask ventilation and intubation.[21] Body mass index alone is not a reliable predictor of a difficult intubation,[22] but anatomic differences in the upper airway in obese patients compared with nonobese patients are associated with difficult intubation.[18] Obese patients can have larger tongues and more redundant oropharyngeal tissue, which can make direct laryngoscopy challenging.[17,21,23] Neck circumference of greater than 40 cm has been shown to be a predictor of difficult intubation.[15]

Cervical spine

Positioning the patient with extension of the upper cervical spine and flexion of the lower cervical spine (sniffing position) or simply extending the neck during direct laryngoscopy optimizes visualization.[24,25] Given the importance of normal cervical spine function in airway management, limitations in cervical spine mobility have implications for a complicated intubation. Karkouti and colleagues[26] showed that impaired atlantoaxial extension is predictive of a difficult intubation. Patients with cervical spine disease have a higher rate of difficult intubation compared with their normal counterparts.[27,28] In addition, large cervical osteophytes can obstruct visualization of the glottis during direct laryngoscopy. The use of videolaryngoscopes or glide scopes can help obtain laryngoscopic visualization in patients with restricted neck movement.[14]

Neck mass/goiter

Previous studies suggested that goiter with tracheal deviation constituted a factor of difficulty during direct laryngoscopy.[29] Mallat and colleagues[30] confirmed that large goiters can increase the risk of poor glottic visualization at direct laryngoscopy but this can be corrected by applying external pressure. Even with marked tracheal deviation, moderate to major difficulty with intubation is not more frequent than in patients without goiters. There was no difference in intubation time between the goiter group and the control group. Gilfillan and colleagues[31] concluded that thyroid patients with a retrosternal goiter, with or without tracheal compression, can be managed with conventional techniques by an experienced anesthesiologist. This management does not preclude the need for multidisciplinary discussion and planning.

Congenital malformations

Patients with congenital malformations have a constellation of disorders, often require multiple surgical procedures, and can be challenging to intubate. There are congenital malformations associated with mandibular hypoplasia, including Treacher Collins, Goldenhar, Crouzon, and Pierre Robin sequence.[32] Pierre Robin sequence is a combination of mandibular hypoplasia, glossoptosis, and cleft palate. These children can have severe airway obstruction necessitating mandibular distraction or tracheostomy tube placement early in life. Klippel-Feil syndrome is a congenital fusion of the cervical vertebrae with severe shortness of the neck and the inability to flex or extend the neck. Patients with Down syndrome have large tongues with small airway diameters and hypotonia, which can make mask ventilation difficult. Care must be taken because patients with Down syndrome can have atlantoaxial instability. If there is a concern for this, the patient should undergo flexion extension cervical spine radiographs before intubation. If atlantoaxial instability is identified, extra care should be taken to minimize neck extension during intubation.[33]

Obstructing airway disorder

The presentation of patients with significant obstructing airway disorder is variable depending on the cause of the obstruction. If the obstruction is a slowly progressing problem (eg, tumor growth), the patient may have been compensating for the gradual decline in the airway and the degree of obstruction can be underestimated based on clinical examination. In contrast, a patient with an acute airway obstruction, such as angioedema or infection (supraglottitis), may be maintaining airway patency with considerably more effort and showing signs of respiratory distress. Flexible laryngoscopy and review of recent imaging studies is advisable before airway management. Flexible laryngoscopy is necessary to indicate the extent, location, and nature of the obstructing disorder.[34] It is well tolerated and quick to perform. Supraglottic tumors are associated with failure of initial attempts at intubation.[13]

Physical Examination Findings

The purpose of the physical examination is to detect physical characteristics that may indicate the presence of a difficult airway (**Box 3**). Because the diagnostic accuracy of a single examination finding or bedside assessment test is limited, multiple airway features should be assessed.[3]

Mouth opening

Interincisor distance less than 3 cm is associated with increased difficulty in intubation with direct laryngoscopy.[1,5,10,18,35] Normal jaw opening can be assessed by asking the patient to insert 2 or 3 fingers into the oral cavity in the midline, which estimates an opening of 4 to 6 cm. It is important to distinguish between muscle spasms and joint restriction because muscle spasms may resolve with muscle relaxants. In a patient with trismus secondary to head and neck cancer treatment, there is fibrosis and muscle relaxation is unlikely to significantly improve mouth opening. Use of videolaryngoscopes can help overcome minor limitations

---

Box 3
Physical examination predictors of difficult intubation

Interincisor distance less than 3 cm[1,5]

Mallampati score greater than 3[4]

Thyromental distance less than 3 finger breadths[3,21]

Short, thick neck[15]

Decreased neck range of motion[27]

in mouth opening, but in severe cases nasofiberoptic intubation should be considered.

Thyromental distance

The thyromental distance is the distance from the thyroid notch to the chin when the head is extended, and it estimates the mandibular space.[3,5,7,21] A distance of less than 6 cm, assessed by the distance of 3 fingerbreadths, has been shown as a predictive factor in difficult intubation.[3,21] The diagnostic utility of the thyromental distance is increased when combined with Mallampati score.[21]

Mallampati score

In common clinical practice, the Mallampati score is the most widely used physical examination test but is characterized by a high percentage of false-positive results (**Box 4**).[3] Mallampati score estimates the size of the tongue relative to the oral cavity and assesses mouth opening. A Mallampati score of 3 or 4 has been associated with difficult intubation, but the positive predictive value is 21% to 50%.[1,10,36] The diagnostic utility of the Mallampati score increases when combined with other examination findings.[21]

Jaw protrusion

Limitations in jaw protrusion or excessive overbite can be associated with difficult intubation.[5] The upper lip bite test can be used to evaluate jaw protrusion and the significance of prominent maxillary incisors. Grade 1 is the ability to cover the mucosa of the lip with the lower teeth, grade 2 is partially able to cover the mucosa of the lip with the lower teeth, and grade 3 is inability to bite the upper lip. Grade 3 is associated with difficult direct laryngoscopy.[7] Again, the predictive value of this test alone is low but can be considered in combination with other physical examination findings.

Flexible Laryngoscopy

The flexible fiberoptic laryngoscope is an important tool for preoperative evaluation of a patient with a potentially difficult intubation. If there is a concerning finding on history or physical examination, a flexible fiberoptic examination can directly evaluate laryngeal access.[37] The procedure is well tolerated and performed quickly with only topical nasal anesthetic and decongestant. The fiberoptic laryngoscope provides excellent visualization of the laryngeal structures and can provide a view of the subglottis or proximal trachea. Details regarding distortion in the normal oropharyngeal, hypopharyngeal, or laryngeal anatomy can be obtained. Evaluations for edema, obstructing cervical osteophytes, or other abnormalities of the upper aerodigestive tract are seen. Rosenblatt and colleagues[34] showed that a preoperative endoscopic laryngeal examination affected the planned airway management in 26% of patients. An awake intubation was planned

---

Box 4
Mallampati classification

Grade 1: visible tonsils, tonsillar pillars and uvula

Grade 2: visible uvula, soft palate

Grade 3: visible soft palate only

Grade 4: visible hard palate only

in 44 of the patients; only 16 underwent awake intubation after preoperative flexible laryngoscopy. In addition, 8 patients were found on examination to have significant laryngeal/pharyngeal disorders and underwent an awake intubation when no prior special intubation was originally planned. Although the flexible laryngoscope is a useful tool, it may not always predict difficulty with direct laryngoscopy.

Radiology

When disorders of the upper aerodigestive tract are identified, imaging studies can give additional information to assist in securing an airway. A computed tomography scan can show the location and degree of airway obstruction, as well as distortion of normal anatomy.

MANAGEMENT

When evaluating management options for the difficult airway situation, the anesthesiologist and surgeon must give consideration to aborting the planned procedure, waking the patient, and reassessing airway management options before proceeding. When this is not an option, the team must consider alternative techniques for laryngoscopy, such as the video-assisted GlideScope, placement of an LMA, intubation by fiberoptic laryngoscopy, direct laryngoscopy with an anterior commissure (Hollinger) laryngoscope, or an awake tracheostomy. Contextual issues, such as patient cooperation, availability of additional skilled help, and the clinician's experience, must also be considered in deciding the appropriate strategy.

Plans A, B, C, and D should be established with a complete discussion among the entire team, including anesthesia, surgeon, scrub technician, and circulating nurse. All necessary equipment should be set up and ready for quick and easy access. A time-out to review the plan and ensure the proper setup should be performed before initiating anesthesia. Preemptive briefing of the entire team increases the likelihood of a coordinated and effective response by all involved if tracheal intubation is not successful on the first attempt.[5]

Formulation of Intraoperative Airway Management Plans

When formulating an intraoperative plan for the management of a predicted difficult intubation, there are several decision points to consider. First, a decision of awake or postinduction tracheal intubation should be made. An awake approach has the potential benefit of having the patient maintain airway patency and protect against aspiration of gastric contents or blood during intubation. In determining awake versus postinduction of general anesthesia, clinicians must consider whether, if anesthesia is induced, tracheal intubation will succeed with the chosen technique, and, if tracheal intubation fails, whether oxygenation by face mask or supraglottic device will succeed. Limitations to the awake technique include patient factors, such as intoxication, noncooperation, mental retardation, and pediatric patients.[11] Second, a decision between the use of noninvasive techniques for the initial approach versus planning for a surgical airway should be determined. Third, a decision should be made between preserving spontaneous ventilation during intubation attempts versus paralysis and ablation of spontaneous ventilation during intubation attempts.[4] It is critically important to determine what part of the airway management is going to be problematic and to choose a management plan that specifically addresses that factor (**Box 5**).

<table>
<tr><td colspan="1">Box 5
Predictors of difficult face mask ventilation</td></tr>
</table>

Box 5
Predictors of difficult face mask ventilation

Higher body mass index or weight

Older age

Male sex

Limited mandibular protrusion

Decreased thyromental distance

Beard

Lack of teeth

Snoring/OSA

Data from Kheterpal S, Healy D, Aziz M, et al. Incidence, predictors and outcome of difficult mask ventilation combined with difficult laryngoscopy. Anesthesiology 2013;119:1360–9.

Intubation After Induction of General Anesthesia

Videolaryngoscopes

Videolaryngoscopes can be effective in enabling a view of the larynx and facilitating intubation when direct laryngoscopy has failed or is predicted to fail. Study X[38] showed that a GlideScope can successfully be used as an alternative to awake fiber-optic intubation in certain patients. Use of a videolaryngoscope increases the success of first-time intubation and can be a useful starting technique for a potentially difficult intubation.[38] Predictors for success with videolaryngoscopes are not the same as for traditional direct laryngoscopy. Mallampati, cervical spine limitations, and jaw protrusion are not associated with difficult GlideScope intubation.[39]

Direct laryngoscopy with the anterior commissure laryngoscope

The Hollinger anterior commissure laryngoscope (**Fig. 1**) can be a useful tool for otolaryngologists, particularly when other methods of direct laryngoscopy have failed. This laryngoscope is designed to provide a view of the anterior larynx and can be useful in fixed laryngeal and subglottic lesions where a small cuffless endotracheal tube may be passed under direct visualization. The Hollinger scope accommodates a 5.0 or smaller cuffed endotracheal tube. If a larger endotracheal tube is required, an Eschmann stylet can be passed through the laryngoscope, and the endotracheal tube is passed over the stylet. The Hollinger anterior commissure scope should be

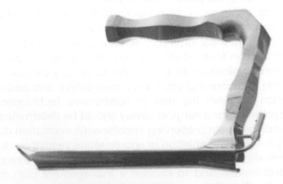

Fig. 1. Hollinger anterior commissure laryngoscope.

set up on the side table before the induction of anesthesia and can be used as a plan B or C if other methods of direct laryngoscopy (Macintosh, Miller blade, videolaryngoscopes) fail to visualize the airway.

Awake Intubation

Awake fiberoptic intubation

When tracheal intubation by direct laryngoscopy is predicted to fail or if induction of anesthesia is likely to result in the inability to mask ventilate a patient, awake fiberoptic intubation should be considered. The ability to maintain spontaneous ventilation and bypass an upper airway obstruction are the main advantages of awake fiberoptic intubation. Morbid obesity, severe trismus, supraglottic mass or edema, and a known history of difficult mask ventilation are indications for awake fiberoptic intubation.[37] It is best performed on patients in the upright position because the tongue does not fall back into the pharynx. Awake fiberoptic intubation is not a good choice for fixed, stenotic lesions of the upper airway, active bleeding obscuring visualization, and complete obstruction of the glottis. For a fixed stenotic lesion of the trachea, perform a direct laryngoscopy and pass the endotracheal tube under visualization using a rigid telescope or rigid bronchoscope. If there is complete obstruction of the glottis, an awake tracheostomy should be performed.

Awake tracheostomy

An awake tracheostomy is an option when intubation through the glottis is not possible. This situation occurs when there is a complete obstructive tumor of the larynx or subglottis, complete laryngeal stenosis, or significant supraglottic edema. An awake tracheostomy tube is performed with no sedation and local anesthesia is used. The patient maintains spontaneous ventilation while the tracheostomy is being performed. Plain lidocaine (1%) is injected into the trachea before entering the airway to minimize coughing. After return of CO_2 is confirmed, generalized anesthesia is immediately administered. An awake tracheostomy tube should not be considered in pediatric patients because the trachea is small and the cartilage is soft and difficult to palpate. In addition, cooperation is not possible. Fixed cervical spine flexion deformity limits access to the neck and makes tracheostomy difficult to perform. Obesity and increased neck circumference result in decreased palpable landmarks and are associated with increased time and difficulty in establishing a secure airway. A large thyroid goiter can also be a limitation to performing an awake tracheostomy and should be evaluated before performing the procedure. Head and neck radiation results in distorted anatomy and loss of palpable landmarks, and can increase the difficulty of performing an awake tracheostomy **(Box 6)**.[40]

Box 6
Predictors of a difficult tracheostomy

Thick/obese neck

Neck radiation

Overlying disorder (tumor, infection)

Displaced airway

Fixed cervical spine flexion deformity

Pediatric patient

---

21. Kim WH, Ahn HJ, Lee CJ, et al. Neck circumference to thyromental distance ratio: a new predictor of difficult intubation in obese patients. Br J Anaesth 2011;106(5): 743–8.
22. Ezrir T, Medalion B, Weisenberg M, et al. Increased body mass index per se is not a predictor of difficult laryngoscopy. Can J Anaesth 2003;50:179–83.
23. Juvin P, Lavaut E, Dupont H, et al. Difficult tracheal intubation is more common in obese than in lean patients. Anesth Analg 2003;97:595–600.
24. Adnet F, Baillard C, Borron SW, et al. Randomized study comparing the sniffing position with simple head extension for laryngoscopic view in elective surgery patients. Anesthesiology 2001;95:836–41.
25. Lewis M, Keramati S, Benumof JL, et al. What is the best way to determine oropharyngeal classification and mandibular space length to predict difficult laryngoscopy? Anesthesiology 1994;81:61–74.
26. Karkouti K, Rose DK, Wigglesworth D, et al. Predicting difficult intubation: a multivariable analysis. Can J Anaesth 2000;47:730–9.
27. Mashour G, Stallmer ML, Kheterpal S, et al. Predictors of difficult intubation in patients with cervical spine limitations. J Neurosurg Anesthesiol 2008;20:110–5.
28. Calder I, Calder J, Crockard HA. Difficult direct laryngoscopy in patients with cervical spine disease. Anaesthesia 1995;50:756–63.
29. Voyagis GS, Kyriakis PK. The effect of goiter on endotracheal intubation. Anesth Analg 1997;84:611–2.
30. Mallat J, Robin A, Pironkov G, et al. Goitre and difficulty of tracheal intubation. Ann Fr Anesth Reanim 2010;29:436–9.
31. Gilfillan N, Ball CM, Myles PS, et al. A cohort and database study of airway management in patients undergoing thyroidectomy for retrosternal goiter. Anaesth Intensive Care 2014;42(6):700–8.
32. Sculerati N, Gottlieb MD, Zimbler MS, et al. Airway management in children with major craniofacial anomalies. Laryngoscope 1998;108:1806–12.
33. Infosino A. Pediatric upper airway and congenital anomalies. Anesthesiol Clin North America 2002;20:747–66.
34. Rosenblatt W, Ianus A, Sukhupragarn W, et al. Preoperative endoscopic airway examination (PEAE) provides superior airway information and may reduce the use of unnecessary awake intubation. Anesth Analg 2011;112:602–7.
35. Rose KD, Cohen MM. The airway: problems and predictions in 18,500. Can J Anaesth 1994;41(5):372–83.
36. Adamus M, Fritscherova S, Hrabalek L, et al. Mallampati test as a predictor of laryngoscopic view. Biomed Pap Med Fac Univ Palacky Olomouc Czech Repub 2010;154:339–44.
37. Osbborn IP, Kleinberger AJ, Gurudult VV. Airway management, emergencies and the difficult airway. In: Levine A, editor. Anesthesiology and otolaryngology. New York: Springer; 2013. p. 115–32.
38. Aziz M, Dillman D, Rongwei F, et al. Comparative effectiveness of the C-Mac video laryngoscope versus direct laryngoscopy in the settings of a predicted difficult airway. Anesthesiology 2012;116:629–36.
39. Diaz-Gomez JL, Satyapriya A, Satyapriya SV, et al. Standard clinical risk factors for difficult laryngoscopy are not independent predictors of intubation success with Glidescope. J Clin Anesth 2011;23:603–10.
40. Maiya B, Smith HL. Failure of tracheostomy under local...plan B? J Laryngol Otol 2006;120(16):882–9.
41. Patel A, Pearce A. Progress in management of the obstructed airway. Anaesthesia 2011;66(2):93–100.

Airway Anesthesia
Theory and Practice

D. John Doyle, MD, PhD[a,b,*]

KEYWORDS

- Airway anesthesia • Airway blocks • Awake intubation • Benzocaine toxicity
- Fiber optic intubation • Lidocaine toxicity • Local anesthesia • Topical anesthesia

KEY POINTS

- Lidocaine is available as a regular solution, a viscous solution, a gel, an ointment, or in a spray can.
- Topicalization is the easiest method for anesthetizing the airway; just spray lidocaine directly onto airway mucosa.
- Needle-based airway blocks are more complicated than noninvasive methods of providing anesthesia to the airway and are usually unnecessary to achieve good airway anesthesia.
- Benzocaine topical anesthesia, although highly effective, is sometimes complicated by methemoglobinemia, the presence of elevated methemoglobin levels within circulating erythrocytes.
- Local anesthetic toxicity with lidocaine, the most commonly used drug for airway anesthesia, can range from tingling, perioral numbness, and paraesthesias to convulsions, coma, and complete cardiorespiratory collapse.

INTRODUCTION

Awake tracheal intubation is commonly used when ordinary intubation (for example, attempting direct laryngoscopy after the induction of general anesthesia) is expected to be difficult or hazardous.[1–8] Possible examples include patients with large glottic tumors, patients with unstable cervical spines, patients known to be difficult to intubate by virtue of previous anesthetic misadventures, and numerous other conditions.[9–15]

This is an updated, reorganized and expanded version of an earlier article published in the 7th Annual Anesthesiology News Guide to Airway Management. August 2014. Available online at: http://anesthesiologynews.com/download/Topicals_ANGAM14_WM.pdf.

[a] Department of General Anesthesiology, Cleveland Clinic Foundation, Abu Dhabi, UAE;
[b] Department of General Anesthesiology, Anesthesiology Institute, Cleveland Clinic Abu Dhabi, PO Box 112412, Abu Dhabi, UAE
* Department of General Anesthesiology, Anesthesiology Institute, Cleveland Clinic Abu Dhabi, PO Box 112412, Abu Dhabi, UAE.
E-mail address: djdoyle@hotmail.com

Regardless of the reason that awake intubation is warranted, however, several underlying principles hold. First, although sedation using drugs such as midazolam, fentanyl, propofol, remifentanil, and dexmedetomidine are undoubtedly useful adjuncts to performing an awake intubation, the "secret recipe" is undoubtedly in obtaining complete anesthesia to the airway structures. With good airway anesthesia, minimal or even no sedation at all can be used, and patient cooperation is much easier to achieve. The purpose of this article is to help make this happen.

MOLECULAR MECHANISMS OF ANESTHESIA

The mechanism by which local anesthetics work has long interested clinicians, and it is customary to comment on this matter in all articles dealing with local anesthesia. Key to this matter is the molecular arrangement common to all local anesthetics (**Fig. 1**).

Until recently, the conventional wisdom is that local anesthetics block voltage-gated sodium channels by binding to a site in the lumen of that channel, thus preventing the flow of current.[16] However, this model has been challenged recently based on the finding that some local anesthetic molecules are too small to fully occlude the sodium channel. This finding has led to an alternative hypothesis that local anesthetics prevent current flow through sodium channels by introducing a positive charge that electrostatically impedes the flow of sodium ions, rather than acting by physical means. For more details, the interested reader is referred to an article by Scheuer.[17]

Fortunately for clinicians, local anesthetics work regardless of how well we understand the underlying molecular mechanisms.

SIX KEY AIRWAY MANAGEMENT DECISIONS

The process begins by making 6 key airway management decisions. The first question asks whether the condition of the airway is so bad that the airway is best managed via a tracheostomy carried out under local anesthesia. Assuming that this is not the case, and additionally, assuming that a supraglottic airway is also inappropriate, let us proceed with the assumption that awake tracheal intubation is desired. Under these assumptions, the second question is then whether one should use the oral as opposed to

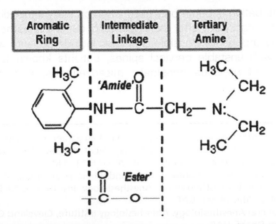

Fig. 1. Most local anesthetics have an aromatic ring on one end, a tertiary amine on the other end, and 1 of 2 forms of an intermediate linkage. This last structural difference (amide vs ester) determines the pathway by which the local anesthetic is metabolized and its potential for allergic reactions. (*From* Becker DE, Reed KL. Local anesthetics: review of pharmacological considerations. Anesth Prog 2012;59(2):90–101; with permission).

the nasal route. In patients with severe trismus, for example, a nasal approach is generally necessary. In addition, the surgeon will sometimes request nasal intubation to make the surgery easier.

The third question is whether one should use needle-based local anesthetic blocks or go with an approach relying entirely on topical anesthesia. Although my preference is for the latter approach, some clinicians favor the use of nerve blocks because of a belief that the chance of local anesthetic toxicity is reduced by virtue of needle-based local anesthetic blocks requiring fewer drugs.

A fourth question is whether glycopyrrolate should be given as an antisialagogue. Although I do this only occasionally, this is a routine practice for a great many clinicians.

The fifth question concerns the appropriate sedation protocol to use. Options include no sedation whatsoever; midazolam, fentanyl, remifentanil dexmedetomidine and propofol in various doses; and other methods (**Table 1**). I often give midazolam, 1 mg, fentanyl, 50 μg, and later propofol, 10 to 20 mg, just before the bronchoscope is introduced.

The sixth question concerns the choice of method of tracheal intubation. Options include fiber-optic intubation, video laryngoscopy, or even regular direct laryngoscopy.

UPPER AIRWAY BLOCKS

For cases in which topical anesthesia is not desired or proven to be ineffective, nerve blocks can be used. Needle blocks are at least relatively contraindicated in patients with coagulopathies or on anticoagulation. Patients should always be aspirated before injecting to help ensure that the needle is not in a blood vessel. Potential complications of these blocks include bleeding, nerve injury, and seizures from intravascular injection.

Glossopharyngeal Block

This block numbs the oropharynx by anesthetizing the glossopharyngeal nerve (ninth cranial nerve), a mixed nerve that provides sensation to the posterior third of the tongue, the vallecula, the anterior surface of the epiglottis (via the lingual branch), the tonsils (via the tonsillar branch), and the pharyngeal walls (via the pharyngeal

Table 1
Commonly used adjunctive medications for awake intubation in adult patients

Medication	Dosage, Route, and Timing	Action	Reversal Agent
Glycopyrrolate	0.2–0.4 mg IV or IM given 15–30 min preprocedure	Antisialagogue	None
Midazolam	0.5–4 mg IV (titrate to effect)	Sedative	Flumazenil
Fentanyl	25–100 μg IV (titrate to effect)	Sedative	Naloxone
Remifentanil	Loading dose: 0.75 μg/kg Infusion: 0.075 μg/kg/min (Cattano et al,[45] 2012)	Sedative	Naloxone
Dexmedetomidine	Loading dose: 1 μg/kg/h over 10-min Infusion: 0.7 μg/kg/h (from product monograph)	Sedative	None

These are guidelines only; smaller does may be appropriate in frail patients, and larger doses may be appropriate in some others.

From Doyle J. Topical and regional anesthesia for awake intubation. 7th Annual Anesthesiology News Guide to Airway Management. 2014. Available at: http://anesthesiologynews.com/download/Topicals_ANGAM14_WM.pdf. Accessed March 23, 2014; with permission.

branch). The glossopharyngeal nerve can be blocked by injecting about 5 mL of local anesthetic (eg, 2% lidocaine) submucosally at the caudal aspect of the posterior tonsillar pillar, where it crosses the palatoglossal arch. Alternatively, the block can be achieved using direct mucosal application via pledgets soaked with local anesthetic (see **Fig. 6**), or even by spraying topical anesthesia onto the above-mentioned region. Some clinicians prefer to avoid needles for this block because it avoids the possibility of seizures from inadvertent injection into the carotid artery. Finally, although this block facilitates intubation by blocking the gag reflex, it is not adequate as a solo technique.

Superior Laryngeal Block

This block numbs the larynx above the vocal cords. The internal branch of the superior laryngeal nerve originates from the superior laryngeal nerve lateral to the greater cornu of the hyoid bone and passes approximately 2 to 4 mm inferior to the greater cornu of the hyoid bone where it pierces the thyrohyoid membrane to innervate the tongue base, the posterior surface of the epiglottis, the aryepiglottic folds, and the arytenoids. To perform this block, the patient is placed in a supine position with the head extended. The hyoid bone is identified and a 25-gauge needle advanced until it makes contact with greater cornu of this structure on the side to be blocked. The needle is then walked off the bone inferiorly and advanced 2 to 3 mm. After a negative aspiration test, 2 to 3 mL of local anesthetic is injected, with an additional 1 to 2 mL administered as the needle is withdrawn. This block is not adequate as a solo technique for airway anesthesia. A video showing the technique is available at http://www.youtube.com/watch?v=8bRlUy7k0LM.

Translaryngeal Block

The translaryngeal block numbs the larynx and trachea below the cords by anesthetizing the recurrent laryngeal nerve, which provides sensation to the trachea and vocal cords. To perform this block, a 5-mL syringe filled with 4% lidocaine and fitted with a 22- or 20-gauge intravenous (IV) catheter is advanced through the cricothyroid membrane until air is aspirated into the syringe. The needle is removed, leaving the IV catheter. Then 4 mL of 4% lidocaine is injected, inducing coughing that scatters the local anesthetic. A video showing the technique is available at http://www.youtube.com/watch?v=I8IF7PjDhnA.

PROCEDURAL MATTERS: 8 STEPS TO AWAKE INTUBATION

The procedure to provide anesthesia via awake intubation involves 8 steps. Note that although the discussion here applies to the use of a fiber optic bronchoscope (**Fig. 2**), the use of a video laryngoscope (**Fig. 3**)[18–23] is another possibility.

The first step in awake intubation is careful preparation: reviewing the clinical issues, checking the equipment, explaining your plan to the patient and clinical team members, applying patient monitors, applying oxygen via nasal cannula, checking the Yankauer and bronchoscope suction systems, checking the patient's IV line, possibly administering glycopyrrolate, and administering sedation if warranted.

The next step is to have the patient gargle 2% viscous lidocaine while positioned upright, administered using a small disposable drinking cup (**Fig. 4**). An alternative to this step involves the use of lidocaine paste (**Fig. 5**). Additionally, some clinicians like to use lidocaine-soaked pledgets as part of the procedure (**Fig. 6**).

This is followed by administering 4% lidocaine to oropharyngeal and glottic structures using an oxygen-driven power sprayer (**Fig. 7**).

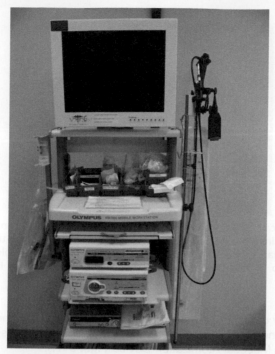

Fig. 2. A fiber optic bronchoscope is the most commonly used device for awake intubation. This model provides a video display that is especially valuable for use in teaching. In addition to airway guides and devices to administer local anesthesia, a bag on the left contains 3 sizes of the i-gel supraglottic airway that can be used as a conduit for intubation, while various kinds of airway catheters hang on the right side of the cart.

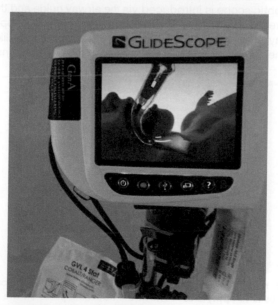

Fig. 3. A video laryngoscope such as the GlideScope (Verathon, Bothell, WA) is sometimes used for awake intubation, for example, when placing special tracheal tubes using a bore too small to admit a bronchoscope.

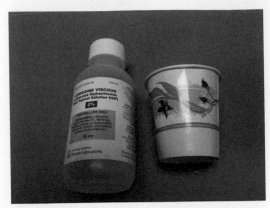

Fig. 4. Viscous lidocaine (Roxane Laboratories, Columbus, OH) at 2% can be given using a small disposable drinking cup. It is gargled, then expectorated; most patients prefer to be sitting up rather than supine for this. In addition, letting the patient hold and control the Yankauer sucker to remove any excess anesthetic or to use after they have had enough can be helpful.

Next, an airway guide is inserted (if fiber optic intubation is planned; **Fig. 8**). Then more 4% lidocaine is administered through the airway guide using the MADgic Laryngo-Tracheal Mucosal Atomization Device (**Figs. 9–11**).

This step is then followed by an immediate preintubation review: confirming that the tracheal tube is taped to the fiber optic scope to prevent slippage, checking that the scope suction is working, checking for good image quality and for correct white balancing, and checking that the propofol is attached to the IV line to ensure ease of starting general anesthesia when the tracheal tube is known to be correctly positioned.

Next, the fiber optic scope is introduced via the airway guide and the epiglottis and the vocal cords are identified. A jaw thrust is sometimes helpful to optimize the alignment of the airway structures. Also, at this point, some clinicians like to administer additional lidocaine via an epidural catheter placed in the biopsy channel of the scope.

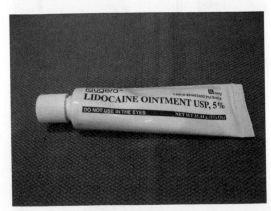

Fig. 5. One popular method of carrying out topical airway anesthesia to oropharyngeal and periglottic structures is to apply 3 to 4 cm of 5% lidocaine paste on the end of a wooden tongue blade, instructing the patient to place the gooey end as far posteriorly in the mouth as possible. Patients should then gently bite on the blade and avoid sucking, letting the paste liquefy onto the airway structures for about 10 minutes.

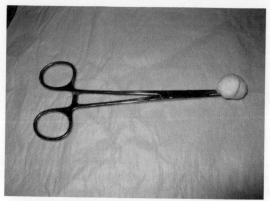

Fig. 6. Apply 4% lidocaine-soaked gauze on a clamp and apply to the pyriform fossa to block the glossopharyngeal nerve and thus the gag reflex (the sensory portion of the glossopharyngeal nerve innervates the posterior third of the tongue, the palatine tonsils, and the mucous membranes of the oropharynx).

Next, the bronchoscope is passed by the cords into the trachea, the carina is identified, the tracheal tube is passed, the tracheal tube cuff is inflated, the patient breathing circuit is connected, and correct tracheal tube positioning should be checked clinically and by capnography.

Finally, anesthesia is induced; both IV and inhalational methods can be used.

NASAL INTUBATION

In cases in which nasal intubation is required, the following additional steps apply after completion of airway topicalization. Patients are instructed to compare their nasal airflow while alternately breathing through the right and left nostril. The nostril with the best airflow is the initial choice for nasotracheal intubation. A spray of 4% cocaine is administered to both nostrils using wide cotton pledgets placed with the aid of alligator forceps. Alternately, a combination of 1% phenylephrine and 4% lidocaine may be used in a 50/50 mixture.

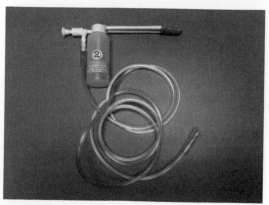

Fig. 7. An oxygen-driven power sprayer can be used to deliver lidocaine to oropharyngeal and glottic structures. Oxygen at 15 liters per minute is used as the gas source. Known as the *EZ-Spray*, this unit is available from Intertex Research, Houston, TX. (EZ-Spray, Intertex Research).

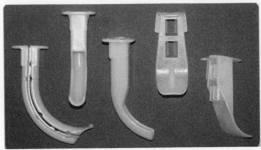

Fig. 8. Airway guides can be useful to facilitate passage of the bronchoscope and tracheal tube. From left to right: Berman, Williams, and Ovassapian airways. (*Courtesy of* Airway Cam, Wayne, PA; with permission).

Although awake nasal intubation is generally completed using fiber optic methods, it can also be achieved via direct or video laryngoscopy.

Fiber Optic Technique

After preparation of the nostrils with one of the above preparations, a well-lubricated endotracheal tube (typically 6.5–7.5 mm inside diameter) is secured to a fiber optic bronchoscope. When the scope has been advanced well into the trachea, the endotracheal tube is railroaded over the scope into position. Twisting may be needed to bypass soft tissue obstruction. The cuff is then inflated, the tube connected to the patient breathing circuit, and correct positioning established by a combination of clinical, capnographic, and fiber optic means.

Technique Using Laryngoscopy

After preparation of the nostrils as discussed earlier, and after testing that the airway is sufficiently well topicalized to allow for awake laryngoscopy, a well-lubricated endotracheal tube previously softened by immersion in hot water is inserted along the floor of the nasal cavity. The tube is directed straight back toward the occiput (not cephalad). Twisting may be needed to bypass soft tissue obstruction. At 6 to 7 cm, one

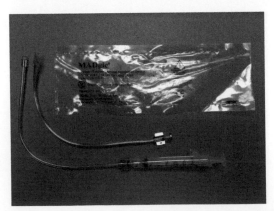

Fig. 9. The malleable LMA MADgic Laryngo-Tracheal Mucosal Atomization Device can be useful to assist in the delivery of topical anesthesia to the periglottic structures (For more information see http://www.teleflex.com/emea/documentLibrary/documents/940716-000001_ LMA-TF-MADgic_1305.pdf). (Teleflex, Wayne, PA).

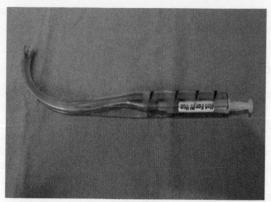

Fig. 10. The malleable LMA MADgic Laryngo-Tracheal Mucosal Atomization Device is also available for use with a disposable rigid guide. (Teleflex, Wayne, PA).

often feels a "give" as the tube passes the nasal choana and enters the nasopharynx. Awake laryngoscopy is then used to visualize the vocal cords and the tip of the endotracheal tube. Using Magill forceps held in the right hand, the endotracheal tube is advanced into the larynx when direct laryngoscopy is used. When video laryngoscopy is used, Boedeker (curved) intubation forceps should be used instead of Magill forceps, although simple manipulation of the head to match the glottic aperture to the

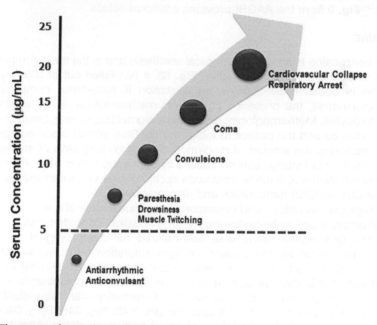

Fig. 11. The types of complications that can occur when local anesthetics are administered in toxic concentrations. In the case of lidocaine, toxicity may occur at blood concentrations exceeding 5 µg/mL. (*From* Becker DE, Reed KL. Local anesthetics: review of pharmacological considerations. Anesth Prog 2012;59(2):90–101; with permission).

trajectory of the tube is sometimes all that is needed. Note that awake nasal intubation using laryngoscopy typically involves more unpleasantness to the patient compared with awake nasal intubation using fiber optic means.

LOCAL ANESTHETIC SAFETY

Although local anesthetics have an impressive history of efficacy and safety in clinical medicine, they are not free of potential adverse effects, especially when given in large doses.[24-31] For plain lidocaine (no added epinephrine), the recommended maximum administered dose is 5 mg/kg or 400 mg for a typical 80-kg man. However, given that this recommendation is intended for cases in which the lidocaine is administered by infiltration (eg, for a plexus block) it would seem that larger doses would be safe in cases in which the drug is mostly gargled and then expectorated. To draw on an analogy, lidocaine doses as large as 35 mg/kg are sometimes given when tumescent anesthesia is used in liposuction procedures.[32] Then again, tumescent anesthesia has been associated with occasional fatal lidocaine toxicity.[33] The types of complications that can occur when local anesthetics are administered in toxic amounts are illustrated in **Fig. 8**.

Guidelines for the management of local anesthetic toxicity have been published by several groups: the American Society of Regional Anesthesia and Pain Medicine (ASRA),[34] the Association of Anaesthetists of Great Britain and Ireland (AAGBI, 2007),[35] and the Resuscitation Council of the United Kingdom. The core principles of management of local anesthetic toxicity involve the termination of seizures, cardiopulmonary support, and use of the lipid rescue protocol where applicable.[36,37] (Because benzodiazepines have limited potential for causing myocardial depression, ASRA recommends these drugs as first-line treatment of local anesthetic–induced seizures).[34] **Fig. 9** from the AAGBI provides additional details.

BENZOCAINE

Although benzocaine is an effective topical anesthetic and is the main component of the popular local anesthetic, Citacaine (**Fig. 12**), it has fallen out of favor in recent years. This is because benzocaine administration is sometimes complicated by methemoglobinemia, the presence of elevated methemoglobin levels within circulating erythrocytes. Methemoglobin, being darkly pigmented, causes blood to appear chocolate colored and the patient to look cyanotic. Dark arterial blood and cyanosis out of proportion to the amount of respiratory distress is suggestive of methemoglobinemia, which, incidentally, can be caused by numerous things other than benzocaine administration (eg, antimalarials such as chloroquine or primaquine, as well as nitrites, nitrates, inhaled nitric oxide, and nitroprusside).

As an example, Sachdeva and colleagues[38] describe a case of a man who underwent transesophageal echocardiography for evaluation of endocarditis in which topical 20% benzocaine spray was administered for oropharyngeal anesthesia. Before the topicalization, the patient's oxygen saturation by pulse oximetry was 97% on room air, but after the benzocaine spray it decreased to 80% despite oxygen administration. Clinically, the patient was cyanotic. Methemoglobinemia was suspected, and arterial blood gas evaluation by CO-oximetry (with the patient on 6 L oxygen via nasal cannula) found the following: pH, 7.42; P_{O_2}, 248; P_{CO_2}, 34; oxygen saturation, 99%; and methemoglobin, 41.8% of total hemoglobin. After treatment with intravenous methylene blue, 2 mg/kg, the cyanosis resolved and a repeat methemoglobin level 2 hours later was 2.8% (Methylene blue acts as a reducing agent via the NADPH methemoglobin reductase pathway.)

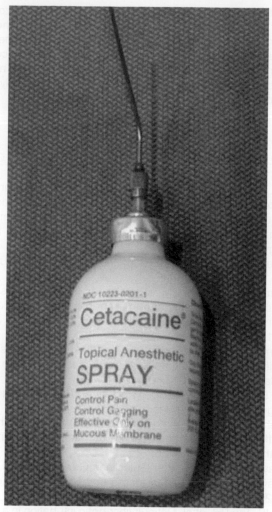

Fig. 12. Cetacaine is a topical anesthetic spray containing benzocaine 14.0%, butamben 2.0%, and tetracaine hydrochloride 2.0%.

Abdel-Aziz and colleagues[39] similarly described the methemoglobinemia with the use of benzocaine spray for awake fiber optic intubation. Another example, Ferraro-Borgida and colleagues[40] described methemoglobinemia in a 34-year-old woman after the perineal application of an over-the-counter cream containing 20% benzocaine.

Finally, clinicians and parents will be interested to know that benzocaine is the active ingredient in many over-the-counter teething pain gels and liquid medications, like Anbesol and Baby Orajel; for the above reasons, the US Food and Drug Administration advises against the use of such products in children younger than 2 years.[41]

FUTURE CONSIDERATIONS/SUMMARY

The safe and effective application of local anesthesia for awake intubation requires attention to several technical details. Patient sedation is less important than ensuring good airway anesthesia. Although lidocaine is preferred over benzocaine, lidocaine toxicity may occur at blood concentrations exceeding 5 μg/mL. Although many clinicians avoid administering more than 5 mg/kg of topical lidocaine (the frequently recommended maximum dose for infiltration), this limit may be conservative in a setting in which much of the drug is not absorbed. Research is needed to clarify this matter; a reasonable starting point would be to systematically measure blood lidocaine levels for various airway topicalization protocols.[31,42–44]

REFERENCES

1. Berkow LC. Strategies for airway management. Best Pract Res Clin Anaesthesiol 2004;18(4):531–48.
2. Apfelbaum JL, Hagberg CA, Caplan RA, et al, American Society of Anesthesiologists Task Force on Management of the Difficult Airway. Practice guidelines for management of the difficult airway: an updated report by the American Society of Anesthesiologists Task Force on Management of the Difficult Airway. Anesthesiology 2013;118(2):251–70.
3. Niven AS, Doerschug KC. Techniques for the difficult airway. Curr Opin Crit Care 2013;19(1):9–15.
4. Law JA, Broemling N, Cooper RM, et al, Canadian Airway Focus Group. The difficult airway with recommendations for management–part 1–difficult tracheal intubation encountered in an unconscious/induced patient. Can J Anaesth 2013; 60(11):1089–118.
5. Law JA, Broemling N, Cooper RM, et al, Canadian Airway Focus Group. The difficult airway with recommendations for management–part 2–the anticipated difficult airway. Can J Anaesth 2013;60(11):1119–38.
6. Wanderer JP, Ehrenfeld JM, Sandberg WS, et al. The changing scope of difficult airway management. Can J Anaesth 2013;60(10):1022–4.
7. Wong DT, Mehta A, Tam AD, et al. A survey of Canadian anesthesiologists' preferences in difficult intubation and "cannot intubate, cannot ventilate" situations. Can J Anaesth 2014;61(8):717–26.
8. Difficult Airway Society Extubation Guidelines Group, Popat M, Mitchell V, et al. Difficult Airway Society Guidelines for the management of tracheal extubation. Anaesthesia 2012;67(3):318–40.
9. Yeh L, Chen HS, Tan PH, et al. Difficult fiber-optic intubation in a patient with giant neck masses: the role of McCoy laryngoscope in elevating compressed laryngeal aperture. Acta Anaesthesiol Taiwan 2013;51(4):180–3.
10. Wood A, Choromanski D, Orlewicz M. Intubation of patients with angioedema: A retrospective study of different methods over three year period. Int J Crit Illn Inj Sci 2013;3(2):108–12.
11. Srivastava D, Dhiraaj S. Airway management of a difficult airway due to prolonged enlarged goiter using loco-sedative technique. Saudi J Anaesth 2013; 7(1):86–9.
12. Kothandan H, Ho VK, Chan YM, et al. Difficult intubation in a patient with vallecular cyst. Singapore Med J 2013;54(3):e62–5.
13. Langeron O, Birenbaum A, Le Saché F, et al. Airway management in obese patient. Minerva Anestesiol 2014;80(3):382–92.
14. Horton CL, Brown CA 3rd, Raja AS. Trauma airway management. J Emerg Med 2014;46(6):814–20.
15. Ghabach MB, Abou Rouphael MA, Roumoulian CE, et al. Airway management in a patient with Le Fort III Fracture. Saudi J Anaesth 2014;8(1):128–30.

16. Butterworth JF 4th, Strichartz GR. Molecular mechanisms of local anesthesia: a review. Anesthesiology 1990;72(4):711–34.
17. Scheuer T. Local anaesthetic block of sodium channels: raising the barrier. J Physiol 2007;581(Pt 2):423.
18. Rothfield KP, Russo SG. Videolaryngoscopy: should it replace direct laryngoscopy? a pro-con debate. J Clin Anesth 2012;24(7):593–7.
19. Curtis R. Awake videolaryngoscopy-assisted tracheal intubation in the morbidly obese. Anaesthesia 2012;67(7):796–7 [author reply: 799].
20. Healy DW, Maties O, Hovord D, et al. A systematic review of the role of videolaryngoscopy in successful orotracheal intubation. BMC Anesthesiol 2012;12:32.
21. Larsson A, Dhonneur G. Videolaryngoscopy: towards a new standard method for tracheal intubation in the ICU? Intensive Care Med 2013;39(12):2220–2.
22. Gu J, Xu K, Ning J, et al. GlideScope-assisted fiberoptic bronchoscope intubation in a patient with severe rheumatoid arthritis. Acta Anaesthesiol Taiwan 2014;52(2):85–7.
23. Agro' FE, Doyle DJ, Vennari M. Use of Glidescope in adults: an overview. Minerva Anestesiol 2015;81(3):342–51.
24. Clapp CR, Poss WB, Cilento BG. Lidocaine toxicity secondary to postoperative bladder instillation in a pediatric patient. Urology 1999;53(6):1228.
25. Moore PA, Hersh EV. Local anesthesia toxicity review revisited. Pediatr Dent 2000;22(1):7–8.
26. Zuberi BF, Shaikh MR, Jatoi NU, et al. Lidocaine toxicity in a student undergoing upper gastrointestinal endoscopy. Gut 2000;46(3):435.
27. Chang YY, Ho CM, Tsai SK. Cardiac arrest after intraurethral administration of lidocaine. J Formos Med Assoc 2005;104(8):605–6.
28. Nishiyama T, Komatsu K. Local anesthetic toxicity in interscalene block: clinical series. Minerva Anestesiol 2010;76(12):1088–90.
29. Menif K, Khaldi A, Bouziri A, et al. Lidocaine toxicity secondary to local anesthesia administered in the community for elective circumcision. Fetal Pediatr Pathol 2011;30(6):359–62.
30. Wolfe JW, Butterworth JF. Local anesthetic systemic toxicity: update on mechanisms and treatment. Curr Opin Anaesthesiol 2011;24(5):561–6.
31. Giordano D, Panini A, Pernice C, et al. Neurologic toxicity of lidocaine during awake intubation in a patient with tongue base abscess. Case report. Am J Otolaryngol 2014;35(1):62–5.
32. Klein JA. Tumescent technique for regional anesthesia permits lidocaine doses of 35 mg/kg for liposuction. J Dermatol Surg Oncol 1990;16(3):248–63.
33. Rao RB, Ely SF, Hoffman RS. Deaths related to liposuction. N Engl J Med 1999;13:1471–5.
34. Neal JM, Bernards CM, Butterworth JF 4th, et al. ASRA practice advisory on local anesthetic systemic toxicity. Reg Anesth Pain Med 2010;35(2):152–61.
35. Picard J, Ward SC, Zumpe R, et al. Guidelines and the adoption of 'lipid rescue' therapy for local anaesthetic toxicity. Anaesthesia 2009;64(2):122–5.
36. Litz RJ, Roessel T, Heller AR, et al. Reversal of central nervous system and cardiac toxicity after local anesthetic intoxication by lipid emulsion injection. Anesth Analg 2008;106(5):1575–7.
37. Leskiw U, Weinberg GL. Lipid resuscitation for local anesthetic toxicity: is it really lifesaving? Curr Opin Anaesthesiol 2009;22(5):667–71.
38. Sachdeva R, Pugeda JG, Casale LR, et al. Benzocaine-induced methemoglobinemia: a potentially fatal complication of transesophageal echocardiography. Tex Heart Inst J 2003;30(4):308–10.

39. Abdel-Aziz S, Hashmi N, Khan S, et al. Methemoglobinemia with the use of benzocaine spray for awake fiberoptic intubation. Middle East J Anesthesiol 2013;22(3):337–40.
40. Ferraro-Borgida MJ, Mulhern SA, DeMeo MO, et al. Methemoglobinemia from perineal application of an anesthetic cream. Ann Emerg Med 1996;27: 785–8.
41. So TY, Farrington E. Topical benzocaine-induced methemoglobinemia in the pediatric population. J Pediatr Health Care 2008;22(6):335–9 [quiz: 340–1].
42. Gulur P, El Saleeby C, Watt LD, et al. Elevated lidocaine serum levels following the use of a needle free device in healthy adult volunteers. Pediatr Emerg Care 2014; 30(5):335–9.
43. Martin KM, Larsen PD, Segal R, et al. Effective nonanatomical endoscopy training produces clinical airway endoscopy proficiency. Anesth Analg 2004;99(3): 938–44.
44. Woodall NM, Harwood RJ, Barker GL. Lidocaine toxicity in volunteer subjects undergoing awake fiberoptic intubation. Anesth Analg 2005;101(2):607 [author reply: 607].
45. Cattano D, Lam NC, Ferrario L, et al. Dexmedetomidine versus Remifentanil for Sedation during Awake Fiberoptic Intubation. Anesthesiology Research and Practice 2012;2012:7. Available at: http://www.hindawi.com/journals/arp/2012/ 753107/.

Obstructive Sleep Apnea, Sleep Disorders, and Perioperative Considerations

Tracey L. Stierer, MD[a,b,*]

KEYWORDS

- Obstructive sleep apnea • Difficult airway • Perioperative • Postoperative
- Monitoring

KEY POINTS

- Patients with obstructive sleep apnea (OSA) are at risk for difficult mask ventilation and tracheal intubation.
- Most patients with OSA do not have a formal diagnosis.
- Identification of patients at risk for OSA may have safety implications in the perioperative period.
- Questionnaire tools can aid in the prediction of the presence of OSA; however, polysomnography is the gold standard test to diagnose the disorder.

INTRODUCTION

Of all the sleep disorders, obstructive sleep apnea (OSA) is the most likely to cause concern for those responsible for managing the airway during the perioperative period. Highly prevalent in the general population, OSA affects 4% and 2% of middle-aged men and women, respectively.[1] OSA has been associated with a number of co-morbidities including cardiovascular disease, arrhythmia, stroke, obesity, metabolic syndrome, insulin resistance, and depression.[2] Untreated, OSA can lead to uncontrolled hypertension, heart failure, and premature death.[3] It has long been recognized that anesthesia and airway manipulation in the patient with OSA can present unique challenges with respect to mask ventilation, tracheal intubation, and

The author has no disclosures.

[a] Anesthesiology and Critical Care Medicine, Johns Hopkins Medicine, 601 North Caroline Street, Baltimore, MD 21287-0712, USA; [b] Otolaryngology, Head and Neck Surgery, Johns Hopkins Medicine, 601 North Caroline Street, Baltimore, MD 21287-0712, USA

* Otolaryngology, Head and Neck Surgery, Johns Hopkins Medicine, 601 North Caroline Street, Baltimore, MD 21287-0712.

E-mail address: tstiere@jhmi.edu

Anesthesiology Clin 33 (2015) 305–314
http://dx.doi.org/10.1016/j.anclin.2015.02.003
1932-2275/15/$ – see front matter © 2015 Elsevier Inc. All rights reserved.

anesthesiology.theclinics.com

postextubation ventilation.[4] Increased airway collapsibility and sensitivity to central nervous system depressants add to the complexity encountered in the perioperative management of the OSA patient. When the patient with a formal diagnosis of OSA presents for an elective surgical procedure, there is sufficient time to prepare for the possibility of a difficult airway, and to discuss with the surgeon and patient a perioperative plan tailored to mitigate the risk of adverse cardiorespiratory events. However, it is known that most patients with OSA have not yet received a formal diagnosis. In some studies, it is suggested that 80% to 90% of patients with OSA remain undiagnosed.[5]

There is growing evidence that early identification of patients at risk for OSA and implementation of strategies to decrease perioperative respiratory depression may alter outcomes.[6] This article examines the available literature as well as current opinion and recommendations for the perioperative management of the patient at risk of OSA.

SYMPTOMS

OSA is characterized by the repetitive partial or complete collapse of the upper airway during sleep.[7] These obstructive events may be accompanied by decreases in oxyhemoglobin saturation and subsequently lead to brief arousals and sleep fragmentation. Patients with OSA may admit to snoring, awaking gasping or choking, and excessive daytime fatigue or sleepiness. Bed partners will often report witnessing the patient's apnea, as well as his or her intermittent snoring and restless sleep. Although the chief complaint of the OSA patient who presents to a sleep disorder clinic is frequently excessive daytime somnolence, the visit may also be at the insistence of the bed partner whose sleep may be equally disrupted by the patient's loud snoring. OSA syndrome (OSAS) is the combination of the presence of OSA coupled with reported clinical sequelae of daytime fatigue.

EPIDEMIOLOGY

Relatively rare in young women, OSAS occurs more commonly in middle-aged men than women with a 3 to 1 or 4 to 1 ratio.[1] This ratio changes, for reasons poorly understood, with hormonal changes that occur when women reach postmenopausal age. With increases in testosterone and decreases in estrogen and progesterone, the risk of OSA for women after menopause becomes equal to that of men.[8] Furthermore, the incidence of OSA increases substantially with age regardless of gender.[9] Reports of familial predisposition to OSA or clustering of symptoms has been described not only with regard to craniofacial morphology and syndromic facies, but also in those with isolated polysomnographic evidence of sleep-related breathing disorders.[10]

African Americans younger than 30 years old, and south Asians have also been shown in some studies to be more prone to OSA than their Caucasian age- and body mass index (BMI)-matched counterparts.[11,12]

RISK FACTORS

Obesity is the most consistently recognized predisposing factor for OSA. The prevalence of OSA in the morbidly obese population has been reported to be as high as 70%.[13] Increased neck circumference has been associated with OSA, as has increased waist hip ratio and central truncal obesity, which is frequently seen in patients suffering from metabolic syndrome.[14–16] Men characteristically have android fat deposition; however, it is prominent in women with polycystic ovarian disease, and it can be seen in patients who are prescribed antiretroviral medications and suffering from lipodystrophy.[17-19] The incidence of OSA has been shown to be increased in both of these populations. Particularly in men, visceral fat has been linked to OSA, whereas in women, total adiposity may be more important in determining risk for OSA.[20] Although intervisceral fat has been associated with the presence of OSA, there are other data that suggest that neck circumference may be a better predictor of the disorder in men.[21] Neck circumferences of 16 inches for a woman and 17 inches for a man are the suggested measurements used by the American Society of Anesthesiology Checklist in determining an individual's risk of OSA.[22]

While highly associated with obesity, OSA can occur, and it is unfortunately frequently overlooked in normal or underweight individuals. There are several bony and soft tissue features of the head and neck that have been implicated in obstruction of the upper airway. Deviation of the nasal septum, tonsillar enlargement, flattened midface, retro- or micrognathia, high arched palate with decreased inter-molar distance, and malpositioned hyoid are just some of the anatomic abnormalities that are capable of causing OSA.[23,24]

PATHOPHYSIOLOGY

A decrease in the cross-sectional area of the airway is responsible for the reduction or cessation of airflow during an apneic or hypopneic episode. Due to anatomic abnormalities, defects in neuromuscular tone, or a combination of both, the upper airway collapses, and inspiratory flow is compromised. Sleep stages are divided into 2 discrete states based on electroencephalographic features and motor activity, non-rapid eye movement (NREM) and rapid eye movement (REM) sleep. Upon initiation of sleep, the activity of pharyngeal dilator muscles responsible for airway patency is decreased. During the REM phase of sleep, accompanying generalized atony further decreases the activity of the pharyngeal and genioglossus muscles, leading to more substantial obstruction of the airway. It has been hypothesized, that unlike their non-OSA counterparts, patients with OSA are unable to mount a neuromuscular response of sufficient strength to overcome airway obstruction.[25] This concept is corroborated by studies that show that electrical stimulation of the genioglossus is capable of correcting airway obstruction.[26] Furthermore, it is unknown whether the abnormal motor activation of the pharyngeal muscles is due to an inherent or acquired deficit, and what role is played by postobstructive microarousal.[27] A systemic illness, OSAS has been associated with an increase in reactive oxygen species as well as serum proinflammatory markers tumor necrosis factor (TNF)-a, interleukin (IL)-1B and IL-6.[28] These cytokines are thought to be partially responsible for the excessive daytime sleepiness experienced by those with the OSAS, and may contribute to the pathogenesis of the disease.

Untreated, repetitive episodes of hypoxemia and hypercarbia lead to a number of physiologic responses. Chronic intermittent hypoxia and associated arousals result in an increase in sympathetic tone and circulating catecholamines, as well as endothelial dysfunction. Chronic oxidative stress promotes vasoconstriction and vascular remodeling, which in turn lead to arterial noncompliance and secondary hypertension. It has been reported that more than 70% of patients with resistant hypertension suffer from OSA.[29] During an obstructive episode, the generation of negative intrathoracic pressure increases afterload, venous return, as well as preload, while the ensuing hypoxia promotes pulmonary artery vasoconstriction and resultant pulmonary hypertension. These perturbations cause distension of the right ventricle, and on echocardiography, the interventricular septum can be seen to be displaced to left during diastole, thereby impairing left ventricular (LV) filling and stroke volume.[30] Myocardial ischemia results from increased LV transmural pressure and myocardial oxygen demand that occur during apnea-related hypoxia and decreased oxygen delivery. This sequence of events can lead to the development of hypertrophy and ultimately, failure.

Patients with OSA are also more likely to develop dysrhythmias, in particular atrial fibrillation (AF), than their non-OSA counterparts. According to the Sleep Heart Health Study, the risk of AF in patients with OSA was found to be 4 times greater than their non-OSA counterparts.[31]

Although the exact pathophysiologic mechanism that links OSA to AF is unknown, multiple theories have been proposed. Atrial stretch that accompanies enlargement, hypoxemia, and changes in autonomic tone may all contribute to the genesis of atrial fibrillation, and data suggest that it is a combination of these factors that induces the dysrhythmia.

DIAGNOSTIC TESTING

Overnight polysomnography (PSG) is the gold standard test used in the diagnosis of OSA as well as many other sleep disorders. Costly, time consuming, and labor intensive, PSG involves the simultaneous recording of multiple physiologic variables while the patient sleeps. A full-montage attended PSG includes electroencephalography, electromyography, electro-oculogram, rhythm, pulse oximetry, nasal airflow, as well as detection of chest and abdominal movement. Microphones may be employed to detect snoring, and cutaneous or end-tidal CO_2 may be measured. Body position is noted and can be an important element in predicting the likelihood of postoperative obstruction especially after procedures in which the patient will recover in the supine or recumbent position.

Scoring variability exists between various laboratories, and there may be night-to-night variability in the scores obtained for an individual patient. According to the American Academy of Sleep Medicine (AASM) Manual for the Scoring of Sleep and Associated Events, an apnea is the complete cessation of airflow for a minimum of 10 seconds (**Fig. 1**).[32] The apnea is scored as obstructive if it meets criteria and is associated with continued or increased inspiratory effort throughout the entire period of absent airflow.

The respiratory event is scored as central if inspiratory effort is absent throughout the entire period of apnea, and an event in which inspiratory effort is absent in the initial portion of the event, but followed by the resumption of inspiratory effort in the second portion is designated as mixed. Criteria used to score a hypopnea are not as straightforward. A hypopnea is scored if the nasal pressure decreases by at least 30% of baseline for a minimum of 10 seconds for at least 90% of the duration of the event, and is associated with at least a 4% decrease in oxyhemoglobin saturation. Alternatively, a 50% or greater reduction of nasal pressure for a minimum of 10 seconds associated with a 3% or greater drop in the oxyhemoglobin saturation has also been used as criteria.

The apnea hypopnea index (AHI) is the total number of apneas and hypopneas recorded during sleep divided by the total sleep time. Excluded from this index are respiratory event-related arousals that do not meet scoring criteria for an apnea or hypopnea, but never the less result in the brief transition to awake state, and thus they may contribute to sleep fragmentation.

Another important polysomnographic index is the oxyhemoglobin nadir as well as the sleep time spent with oxygen saturations below 90% (T90%).

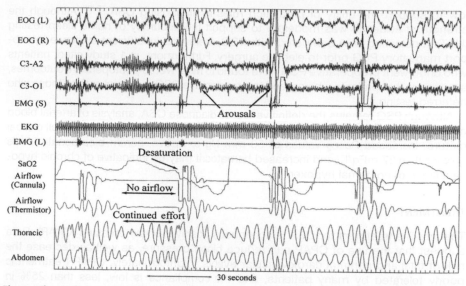

Fig. 1. Channels recorded. Electrooculogram (EOG) from both eyes; electromyogram (EMG) of chin (S) and leg (L); electroencephalogram (EEG) from standard locations C3-A2, C3-O1; electrocardiogram (ECG); oxygen saturation (SaO2); airflow (cannula and thermistor); respiratory effort (thoracic and abdomen).

Acknowledging the previously described criteria may provide clues as to why investigators have experienced difficulty in associating AHI with perioperative outcome. Although apneic or hypopneic episodes must be at least 10 seconds in duration, there can be tremendous variability in duration of each scored event. Likewise the degree of oxyhemoglobin desaturation associated with each event may range from relatively mild to profound.

Whether preoperative polysomnography affects patient outcome remains unclear. In 2006, the American Society of Anesthesiologists (ASA) convened a task force to provide recommendations for the perioperative care of the patient with known or suspected OSA.[22] Faced with a relative paucity of quality data upon which to base recommendation for clinical practice, the task force published a consensus document rooted mainly in consensus of opinion. The practice parameters included a checklist of signs and symptoms that was to be utilized in the determination of presumptive diagnosis of OSA in patients in whom the disorder was suspected. This consensus statement was updated in 2014; however, no changes were made to the recommendations concerning the checklist.[33] In 2011, in response to a public request, a review was performed to examine the relative effectiveness of approaches to screening, diagnosis, and treatment of OSA.[34] Two-hundred thirty-four clinical studies were included in the effort to provide information to aid in discussion with patients and assistance with decision making. Seven key questions were addressed in the report, including the usefulness of screening questionnaires, accuracy of portable home monitoring devices, and utility of preoperative PSG. Several questionnaires have been utilized clinically to predict the presence of OSA. The Berlin Questionnaire, Ward Flemons's Sleep Apnea Clinical Score, the ASA Checklist, and the STOP-Bang Questionnaire are among the prediction models that have used to determine the risk of OSA; however the reviewers concluded that the strength of evidence was low to support the utility of prediction rules in diagnosing OSA.[35–38] Although the strength of evidence was moderate to support the accuracy of home sleep testing (HST) in detecting OSA compared with PSG, there was insufficient evidence to support mandatory PSG prior to elective surgery. Furthermore, in 1 study cited, patients who underwent preoperative PSG were found to have worse postoperative outcomes, suggesting that patients who agreed to preoperative PSG were sicker than those who deferred testing.[37]

Although PSG remains the definitive test to diagnose OSA, analysis of arterial blood gas, serum chemistry, and complete blood count may contribute to the overall clinical picture. Increased $Paco_2$ values of 50 mm Hg or above, serum bicarbonate levels greater than 27 mEq/L, and increased hematocrit may be indicative of chronic hypoventilation or nocturnal hypoxemia.

TREATMENT

The first-line treatment for OSA is continuous positive airway pressure (CPAP). Data suggest that the use of CPAP can reduce blood pressure, as well as decrease the risk of fatal and nonfatal cardiovascular events.[39] Unfortunately, CPAP treatment is poorly tolerated by many patients, and the compliance is low, less than 25% in some studies.[40] Depending on the severity of OSA, alternative treatments options can be considered. Dental appliances that temporarily displace the mandible forward when worn during sleep can alleviate airway obstruction in a subset of patients with mild-to-moderate OSA (AHI <30 events/h). Positional therapy or side sleeping may also be effective for individuals who exhibit a strong positional component to their obstructive episodes on PSG.

Depending on the nature of the airway obstruction, there is a variety of surgical treatment options available ranging from minimally invasive outpatient procedures to more extensive surgeries that may require a stay of several nights in the hospital. The choice of procedure is based upon the site of obstruction, which can be anywhere in the upper airway from the nose to the larynx. Additionally, procedures may be classified as either single- or multilevel; however, there is a lack of quality data addressing the effectiveness of many procedures. As for the single level procedures, both septoplasty and turbinate reduction are common treatments offered to patients who complain of nasal congestion associated with OSA. Uvulopalatopharyngoplasty (UPPP) and tonsillectomy involve the removal of excess tissue as well as strategic placement of sutures in order to increase room in the oropharynx. Although relatively effective at alleviating snoring, the success rate for treatment or cure of OSA is much lower.[41] Hyoid and tongue advancement, soft palate polyester implants (Pillar procedure), as well as base of tongue reduction via radiofrequency waves or direct excision have all been shown to be effective treatments for certain populations of patients with OSA.[42] Among the most effective surgical remedies for OSA are maxillomandibular advancement and tracheostomy.[43] Although technically challenging and potentially painful, expansion of the airway by surgical manipulation of the maxillofacial boney structures has been shown to have a success rate of approximately 90%. Tracheostomy bypasses the upper airway; however, considered an extreme maneuver, the procedure is reserved for the very ill patient, or those who have failed other surgical treatments.

Recently, Woodson and colleagues[44] examined the efficacy of therapeutic upper airway stimulation as part of the Stimulation Treatment for Apnea Reduction (STAR) trial. Patients with a known history of moderate-to-severe OSA who were unable to tolerate CPAP therapy received a stimulation cuff electrode on the submandibular branch of the right hypoglossal nerve. The authors concluded that continuous use of upper airway stimulation (UAS) at night improved breathing and oxygen saturations as well as reducing sleep interruption and daytime sleepiness.

MANAGEMENT

Perioperative management of patients with OSA is aimed at optimization of associated comorbidities, preparation for a difficult airway, aspiration prophylaxis, and avoidance of factors that contribute to respiratory depression. In 2012, the Joint Commission issued a sentinel event alert advising that all hospitalized patients be screened for risk of respiratory depression and presence of OSA; unfortunately, there is variable compliance among institutions with this recommendation.[45] The choice of surgical venue, the decision to perform a procedure on an ambulatory or inpatient basis, and the postoperative monitoring requirements for the patient with OSA remain sources of discussion and controversy. Guidance from the original practice parameters issued by the ASA in 2006 recommended against discharge of the OSA patient undergoing any ambulatory procedure except those performed under straight local anesthesia on the day of surgery.[22] Although these guidelines were updated in 2014, the task force did not feel the need to amend any of their prior recommendations.[33] Subsequent data from Johns Hopkins challenged this position with a study that suggested that ambulatory surgery for appropriately selected patients was not associated with unplanned admission, readmission, or serious respiratory or cardiovascular adverse events.[46] In 2012, The Society for Ambulatory Anesthesia issued a consensus statement addressing the appropriate patient selection for adult patients scheduled for ambulatory surgical procedures.[47] In this document, the authors advised that OSA patients with controlled comorbidities may be reasonable candidates for ambulatory procedures if their pain can be appropriately managed with minimal or no postoperative opioids.

The optimal duration and level of postoperative monitoring of the OSA patient with poorly controlled comorbidities, or for those scheduled for inpatient surgical procedures have not yet been defined. There is little safety advantage gained by overnight admission of the OSA patient to an unmonitored general ward instead of home with regard to prevention of respiratory depression or arrest. Continuous pulse oximetry has been shown to be of value, but only when central monitoring and reliable alert systems are employed.[48,49] Furthermore, pulse oximetry is a late indicator of hypoventilation in the presence of supplemental oxygen. Although there is general agreement that patients with OSA would benefit from monitoring of ventilation, there are few data to guide the best choice of parameter or type of technology. End tidal carbon dioxide (ETCO2), while used frequently to monitor ventilation in nonintubated patients undergoing procedural sedation, may be difficult to use on the general care ward, as patients may preferentially mouth breathe or remove monitoring apparatus in the night. This may lead to alarm fatigue, disabling of alarms, and a potential false sense of security. Recent technological advances have been aimed at the development of a noncumbersome sensor with easy-to-interpret data that would detect changes in ventilation status in hospitalized patients; however, insufficient data exist to recommend the routine use of any of these devices.

SUMMARY/FUTURE CONSIDERATIONS

Data to guide the perioperative identification and clinical management of the patient at risk of OSA are rapidly emerging; however, many questions remain unanswered. PSG, the standard test used to diagnose the presence of OSA, may not be convenient or available in all hospitals, and many patients may not be interested in the time, effort, and potential cost associated with obtaining the study. Although there are several questionnaire tools that have been used to predict the presence of OSA in undiagnosed patients, issues pertaining to specificity and sensitivity make choosing a threshold for risk score difficult. Additionally, the phenotype of the patient at risk for OSA who may suffer from postoperative adverse event has not been defined. With limited monitored beds available in most hospitals, it is difficult to determine which patients should be triaged to or would benefit most from extended postoperative monitoring for respiratory compromise. Further studies are needed to help guide clinical decision making in the perioperative management of patients at risk of OSA.

REFERENCES

1. Young T, Palta M, Dempsey J, et al. The occurrence of sleep disordered breathing among middle aged adults. N Engl J Med 1993;328(17):1230–5.
2. Xie W, Zheng F, Song X. Obstructive sleep apnea and serious adverse outcomes in patients with cardiovascular and cerebrovascular disease: a PRISMA-compliant systematic review and meta-analysis. Medicine 2014; 93(29):e336.
3. Costa C, Santos B, Severino D, et al. Obstructive sleep apnea syndrome: an important piece in the puzzle of cardiovascular risk factors. Clin Investig Arterioscler 2014. [Epub ahead of print].
4. Toshniwal G, McKelvey GM, Wang H. STOP-Bang and prediction of difficult airway in obese patients. J Clin Anesth 2014;26(5):360–7.
5. Young T, Evans L, Finn L, et al. Estimation of the clinically diagnosed proportion of sleep apnea syndrome in middle-aged men and women. Sleep 1997;20(9): 705–6.
6. Mutter TC, Chateau D, Moffatt M, et al. A matched cohort study of postoperative outcomes in obstructive sleep apnea: could preoperative diagnosis and treatment prevent complications? Anesthesiology 2014;121(4):707–18.
7. American Academy of Sleep Medicine. International classification of sleep disorders: diagnostic and coding manual. 2nd edition. Westchester (IL): American Academy of Sleep Medicine; 2005.
8. Bixler EO, Vgontzas AN, Lin HM, et al. Prevalence of sleep-disordered breathing in women: effects of gender. Am J Respir Crit Care Med 2001;163:608–13.
9. Bixler EO, Vgontzas AN, Ten Have T, et al. Effects of age on sleep apnea in men: I.prevalence and severity. Am J Respir Crit Care Med 1998;157:144–8.
10. Campana L, Eckert DJ, Patel SR, et al. Pathophysiology & genetics of obstructive sleep apnoea. Indian J Med Res 2010;13:176–87.
11. Sutherland K, Lee RW, Cistulli PA. Obesity and craniofacial structure as risk factors for obstructive sleep apnoea: impact of ethnicity. Respirology 2012;17(2): 213–22.
12. Leong WB, Arora T, Jenkinson D, et al. The prevalence and severity of obstructive sleep apnea in severe obesity: the impact of ethnicity. J Clin Sleep Med 2013; 9(9):853–8.
13. Lopez PP, Stefan B, Schulman CI, et al. Prevalence of sleep apnea in morbidly obese patients who present for weight loss surgery evaluation: more evidence for routine screening for OSA before weight loss surgery. Am Surg 2008;74: 834–8.
14. Cowan DC, Allardice G, Macfarlane D, et al. Predicting sleep disordered breathing in outpatients with suspected OSA. BMJ Open 2014;4(4):e004519.

15. Deng X, Gu W, Li Y, et al. Age-group-specific associations between the severity of obstructive sleep apnea and relevant risk factors in male and female patients. PLoS One 2014;9(9):e107380.
16. Seetho IW, Wilding JP. Sleep-disordered breathing, type 2 diabetes and the metabolic syndrome. Chron Respir Dis 2014;11(4):257–75.
17. Walker GE, Marzullo P, Ricotti R, et al. The pathophysiology of abdominal adipose tissue depots in health and disease. Horm Mol Biol Clin Investig 2014;19(1):57–74.
18. Nandalike K, Agarwal C, Strauss T, et al. Sleep and cardiometabolic function in obese adolescent girls with polycystic ovary syndrome. Sleep Med 2012; 13(10):1307–12.
19. Lo Re V 3rd, Schutte-Rodin S, Kostman JR. Obstructive sleep apnoea among HIV patients. Int J STD AIDS 2006;17(9):614–20.
20. Kritikou I, Basta M, Tappouni R, et al. Sleep apnoea and visceral adiposity in middle-aged male and female subjects. Eur Respir J 2013;41(3):601–9.
21. Lim YH, Choi J, Kim KR, et al. Sex-specific characteristics of anthropometry in patients with obstructive sleep apnea: neck circumference and waist-hip ratio. Ann Otol Rhinol Laryngol 2014 Jul;123(7):517–23.
22. American Society of Anesthesiologists. Practice guidelines for the perioperative management of patients with obstructive sleep apnea: a report by the American Society of Anesthesiologists Task Force on perioperative management of patients with obstructive sleep apnea. Anesthesiology 2006;104:1081–93.
23. Georgalas C. The role of the nose in snoring and obstructive sleep apnoea: an update. Eur Arch Otorhinolaryngol 2011;268(9):1365–73.
24. S1 Shi, Xia Y, Zhu M, et al. Characterization of upper airway obstruction by fiber-optic nasolaryngoscopy and MRI in preoperative OSAHS patients. ORL J Otorhinolaryngol Relat Spec 2014;76(6):321–8.
25. McGinley BM, Schwartz AR, Schneider H, et al. Upper airway neuromuscular compensation during sleep is defective in obstructive sleep apnea. J Appl Physiol (1985) 2008;105(1):197–205.
26. Eastwood PR, Barnes M, Walsh JH, et al. Treating obstructive sleep apnea with hypoglossal nerve stimulation. Sleep 2011;34(11):1479–86.
27. Fogel RB, Trinder J, White DP, et al. The effect of sleep onset on upper airway muscle activity in patients with sleep apnoea versus controls. J Physiol 2005; 564(Pt 2):549–62.
28. Nadeem R, Molnar J, Madbouly EM, et al. Serum inflammatory markers in obstructive sleep apnea: a meta-analysis. J Clin Sleep Med 2013;9(10):1003–11.
29. Logan AG, Perlikowski SM, Mente A, et al. High prevalence of unrecognized sleep apnea in drug-resistant hypertension. J Hypertens 2001;19(12):2271–7.
30. Kasai T. Sleep apnea and heart failure. J Cardiol 2012;60(2):78–85.
31. Mehra R, Benjamin EJ, Shahar E, et al. Sleep heart health study association of nocturnal arrhythmias with sleep-disordered breathing: the sleep heart health study. Am J Respir Crit Care Med 2006;173(8):910–6.
32. Iber C, Ancoli-Israel S, Chesson A, et al. SF for the American Academy of Sleep Medicine. The AASM manual for the scoring of sleep and associated events: rules, terminology and technical specifications. 1st edition. Westchester (IL): American Academy of Sleep Medicine; 2007.
33. American Society of Anesthesiologists Task Force on Perioperative Management of patients with obstructive sleep apnea. Practice guidelines for the perioperative management of patients with obstructive sleep apnea: an updated report by the American Society of Anesthesiologists Task Force on Perioperative Management of patients with obstructive sleep apnea. Anesthesiology 2014;120(2):268–86.

ANATOMY
Vertebral and Ligamentous Anatomy

The normal cervical spine is composed of 7 vertebrae, the intervertebral discs, and numerous ligaments. The C1 (atlas) and C2 (axis) vertebrae support the weight of the skull. The atlanto-occipital and atlantoaxial joints, as well as the C5-C7 vertebrae are the articular surfaces most involved in head flexion/extension. Lateral rotation involves primarily the atlantoaxis, and can approach 40° from midline in either direction.

The extent of flexion/extension and rotation are regulated and supported by the various ligaments. The posterior column ligaments include the supraspinous, interspinous, and ligamentum flavum, which prevent overflexion of the neck. The anterior column provides stability during extension and includes the anterior and posterior longitudinal ligaments, as well as the transverse, alar, and apical ligaments, which secure the odontoid process of C2 to the anterior arch of C1. This ligamentous attachment is particularly important in limiting translation of the atlantoaxial joint. The facet joints, intervertebral discs, and the intertransverse, interspinous, and supraspinous ligaments contribute to stability of the lower cervical spine.

Pathogenesis of Secondary Injury

Blunt force trauma to the head can cause numerous perturbations of normal bony or ligamentous anatomy of the atlantoaxis, atlanto-occipital complex, and the subaxial vertebrae, depending on the vector of force applied.[1] Even in the absence of a fracture, the spine may still be unstable as a result of a ligamentous injury. An unstable spinal column results in a spinal canal that can change in size with cervical motion.[2] In the intact cervical spine, the extra space of the spinal canal provides a buffer, which prevents excessive contact between the bony elements and the spinal cord. Without this buffer, secondary injury may occur with motion and compression of the spinal cord, leading to negative neurologic outcomes.

EPIDEMIOLOGY
Cervical Spine Trauma

Cervical spine instability may be broadly categorized as congenital or acquired. Of the acquired instabilities, traumatic cervical spine injury (CSI) is the most common. The United States has the highest prevalence of traumatic spinal cord injury in the world, at 908 per million.[3] Blunt trauma is associated with a 1% to 3% incidence of CSI. In a recent analysis of more than 250,000 trauma admissions over a 21-year period, significant predictors of CSI included mechanism of injury (fall, sports injury, motor vehicle related), age less than 30 years, and male sex.[4] A Glasgow Coma Scale score of less than 8 or unconsciousness, obvious facial or head trauma, hypotension, and a focal neurologic deficit have all been associated with up to a 58-fold increase in the odds of a concomitant CSI.[5–7]

The second cervical vertebra is the most common level of injury, followed by fractures of the 2 lowest cervical vertebrae (C6 and C7). A recent analysis found that nearly one-third of all injuries were considered clinically insignificant in that they did not produce instability.[8] Injuries to the upper cervical spine are responsible for up to 80% of mortality related to cervical spine trauma.[9,10]

Nontraumatic Cervical Spine Instability

Acquired instability of the cervical spine is commonly the result of arthritic degeneration.[11] A high proportion of patients with rheumatoid arthritis have cervical neck pain or radicular symptoms with radiographic evidence of atlantoaxial instability. The incidence has decreased since the implementation of disease-modifying antirheumatic drugs and biologics.[12] Ankylosing spondylitis and other spondyloarthropathies have been associated with decreased cervical range of motion, kyphotic deformity, and poor compliance resulting in fracture after minimal neck extension or seemingly trivial trauma.[13,14] These are often severe injuries owing to the localization of extreme displacement at the fracture site.[15] In addition, pathologic fractures related to underlying malignancy or infection may affect the cervical spine by direct compression from mass, or by bony/ligamentous instability.

Several genetic conditions are associated with abnormal cervical spine development and ligamentous laxity, and have been recently reviewed elsewhere **(Table 1)**.[16] Abnormal bony development can result in small or abnormal vertebrae resulting in an unstable articular surface and cord impingement with movement, or a fixed decreased spinal canal diameter. Because of the heterogeneous constellation of physical findings with various congenital syndromes, the degree of impingement on the spinal cord and risk of damage vary. Patients with congenital cervical spine instability require careful individual evaluation.

EVALUATION
Screening for Low-risk Patients

Controversy remains over which patients with trauma may be considered low risk for CSI, and which require advanced imaging. The National Emergency X-radiography Utilization Study (NEXUS) was designed to identify clinical criteria that put patients at low risk for CSI.[17] The 5 criteria that must be met are no midline cervical tenderness, no focal neurologic deficit, normal alertness, no intoxication, and no painful distracting injury. The Canadian CT Head and Cervical Spine Study Group evaluated a different decision tool with only 3 questions to predict CSI in low-risk patients: is there any high-risk factor present that mandates radiography, are there low-risk factors that would allow a safe assessment of range of motion, and is the patient able to actively rotate the neck to the right and left 45°.[18] The NEXUS and Canadian C-spine Rule have been prospectively compared and the Canadian C-spine Rule was superior in both sensitivity and specificity.[19,20] In clinical practice the implementation of these guidelines are variable and may combine aspects of both criteria.

Table 1	
Syndromes associated with cervical spine instability and common anatomic abnormalities observed	
Syndrome	**Abnormality**
Down syndrome	C1-C2 and occipital-C1 transverse ligamentous laxity
22q11.2 deletion	C1 absence or hypoplasia, C2-C3 fusion
Pseudoachondroplasia	Odontoid hypoplasia
Mucopolysaccharidoses	Odontoid hypoplasia with glycosaminoglycan deposition in the dens, ligaments lax, narrow spinal canal
Spondyloepiphyseal dysplasia congenita	Odontoid hypoplasia, small C1 canal opening, ligamentous laxity
Goldenhar syndrome	C1-C2 instability, occiput-atlas fusion, incomplete vertebral ring
Fibrodysplasia ossificans and Klippel-Feil syndrome	Odontoid hypoplasia, cervical ankylosis

Radiographic Clearance

Advanced radiographic imaging is indicated in an unconscious patient with suspected cervical spine instability, or a patient who does not meet NEXUS on C-Spine Rule criteria. Plain films cannot evaluate soft tissue swelling in the lateral view, and have particularly poor sensitivity for upper cervical fractures or involvement of the odontoid.[21] Helical computed tomography (CT) imaging provides significantly increased sensitivity and specificity.[22] CT is unable to identify ligamentous injury directly; however, ligamentous injury can be suggested by observing translation/angulation and rotational abnormalities of the vertebrae. MRI has been combined with CT for optimal radiographic clearance, and ligamentous injuries not identified on CT have been identified on subsequent MRI.[23] MRI has a high detection rate for soft tissue and ligamentous injuries, which may or may not be clinically significant.[24–26]

Although most patients with blunt trauma do not have a CSI, a missed injury can lead to serious outcomes. For this reason, at-risk patients receive spinal immobilization and potentially advanced imaging if indicated.[27] Clearance of the cervical spine, performed by specialized medical professionals, involves consideration of the mechanism of injury; physical examination in an alert, nonaltered patient without distracting injuries; and potentially advanced imaging. Until the cervical spine can be cleared, the patient should remain immobilized.

Immobilization

The goals of spinal immobilization after injury are to maintain the spine in a normal physiologic alignment and to protect the spinal cord from secondary injury.[28] Delayed immobilization associated with missed or delayed diagnosis is thought to be the leading cause of secondary neurologic injury. A rigid cervical collar combined with lateral sandbags and tape has been shown as the most immobilizing combination, but is overly restrictive for prolonged use.[24,29] Mouth opening is significantly reduced by semirigid collars and may cause difficult laryngoscopy.[30]

AIRWAY MANAGEMENT

Airway management of an unstable CSI requires consideration of difficult airway risk factors, patient factors, provider experience, and potential for secondary neurologic injury with positioning, ventilation, and laryngoscopy. All airway maneuvers and airway management devices result in varying degrees of cervical motion, even of the immobilized spine.

Basic Airway Maneuvers

Anatomically, the jaw-thrust and sniffing positions that facilitate ventilation and laryngoscopy also apply forces to the cervical spine that result in movement. Whether these forces are significant or the movement severe enough to compromise the spinal cord depends on the type/degree of injury. In a study of fresh cadavers, a chin lift and jaw thrust resulted in disc space expansion of greater than 5 mm at the site of an experimental injury,[31] and mask ventilation alone resulted in up to 3 mm of cervical spine displacement.[32] The use of cricoid pressure has not been shown to result in clinically significant cervical spine movement in recent studies.[33,34]

Immobilization During Airway Management

To facilitate mouth opening and access the airway, the cervical collar must often be removed while maintaining immobilization. Airway management of patients in cervical collars may be met with higher rates of first-attempt failure, even with video laryngoscopy.[35] Manual in-line stabilization (MILS) has been used for immobilization after the cervical collar is removed and is performed by a second provider with 2 hands maintaining the cervical spine and head in a neutral position, limiting movement during airway manipulation. There is no randomized trial evaluating the use of MILS during airway management for reducing the incidence of neurologic injury,[36,37] but lack of MILS during airway management has been associated with catastrophic neurologic deterioration.[38–40]

During direct laryngoscopy (DL) and other airway maneuvers, MILS has been shown to limit head extension[41] and decrease vertebral subluxation and angulation in a cadaveric model of C5-C6 transection.[42] Nonetheless, MILS has been shown to either fail to prevent or slightly increase subluxation at multiple cervical vertebral levels after experimental destabilization.[43,44] Because of the nature of intubation while maintaining MILS, it has been associated with poor laryngoscopic view, increased time to intubation, and decreased mouth opening.[45] Despite its potential drawbacks, MILS is a simple and easily performed method to limit motion and has been widely accepted during airway management for suspected unstable CSI over the past 3 decades,[46] and there have been few if any reports of neurologic deterioration with its use.[39] MILS should be used to provide spinal immobilization during airway management of a potentially unstable cervical spine to ideally prevent secondary neurologic injury.

Airway Devices

Implementation of any airway device causes some degree of cervical spine motion. The choice of airway device for laryngoscopy depends on several patient and environmental factors. In an emergency, advanced airway devices may not be expediently available. In patients with additional predictors of a difficult airway, or for the elective management of a patient with subacute cervical spine instability, a more controlled approach is warranted. In patients with a full stomach, or active vomiting, time taken to secure the airway may be an important factor that alters patient outcome. The relative pros and cons of each of the commonly used devices are listed in **Table 2**.

Direct Laryngoscopy

A recent retrospective review measuring the success of first-attempt intubation with DL in patients with trauma found a high rate of success and safety.[47] However, there remains significant concern among clinicians about neurologic injury associated with its use. There is some anatomic reason for concern; in normal patients under general anesthesia and without MILS, DL produces extension of each vertebral segment, most concentrated at the occipital-C1 and C1-C2 segments.[48] In injured spine models, Donaldson and colleagues[33] showed a decreased space available for the spinal cord with DL and airway maneuvers.

Degree of cervical movement between blade types has been studied with conflicting evidence. The Miller blade had significantly less movement in a study comparing it with a Macintosh or McCoy hinged blade in immobilized cadavers with C5-C6 transection modeled injury. The degree of cervical extension during laryngoscopy was also evaluated between Macintosh and Miller blades in healthy, not immobilized volunteers. The investigators found a statistically significant but quantitatively small decrease in cervical extension that was thought to be clinically insignificant.[49]

Several case reports have been published and summarized describing worsening neurologic injury after laryngoscopy with and without MILS.[50] These cases generally describe and indicate that although neurologic injury is possible, it is difficult to temporally associate with airway management, and that several confounding factors are typically present.[39] At present it remains unknown whether DL is definitively

Table 2
Airway devices and their benefits and drawbacks for use in patients with potential cervical spine instability

Device	Benefits	Drawbacks
DL	Requires less training than other techniques Most rapid means of securing airway	May be more challenging with immobilization Cervical spine motion occurs even with immobilization
Videolaryngoscopy	Improved view of vocal cords Widely available and minimal training required	Cervical spine motion still occurs despite indirect view Increased time to intubation
Lighted/optical stylets	Less cervical motion than DL May be faster than fiberoptic intubation	Light wand is a blind technique May be challenging; increased risk of failure
Supraglottic airway devices	LMA remains a part of the difficult airway algorithm for cannot-intubate, cannot-ventilate situations	Pressure applied to cervical vertebrae, enough to displace cervical spine posteriorly High rate of failure as a conduit for blind intubation Injuries reported with use
Awake fiberoptic intubation	Least amount of cervical spine motion Allows postintubation neurologic examination	Technically challenging Advanced airway equipment and setup required Prolonged time to intubation compared with other methods Awake technique requires plan for sedation, anesthesia of the airway, and patient cooperation Blood/secretions in airway may obscure view

Abbreviation: LMA, laryngeal mask airway.

associated with an increase in the odds of neurologic deterioration. DL with MILS is perhaps the most rapid and reliable way to secure the airway when limited resources are available, and has been shown to be a safe technique.[51] A survey of clinical practice patterns in the prevideolaryngoscope era indicated that DL was the preferred technique for airway management of unstable or apneic patients with a potential CSI.[52]

Rigid Video Laryngoscopy

Video laryngoscopes have become widely available in the past 10 years and are increasingly used for patients with CSI.[53,54] In practice, multiple types of videolaryngoscopy have been shown to provide improved glottic view even with neck immobilization, but to also require significantly more time to secure the airway.[55,56] Laryngoscopy with a GlideScope took 62% longer than with the Macintosh blade in one recent study of uninjured volunteers.[57]

The biomechanics of videolaryngoscopy are less clear. The theoretic benefit was once thought to be a reduction in the forces exerted on the cervical spine, because of the indirect view of the vocal cords obtained. However, one recent comparison of videolaryngoscopy with DL found that cervical spine motion during endotracheal intubation was not directly proportional to force. The investigators concluded that low-force laryngoscopes could not be assumed to result in proportionally lower cervical spine motion.[58] However, without the use of MILS, less cervical extension has been documented with various scopes compared with DL.[54]

Studies of cervical motion of healthy volunteers with MILS have mixed results.[54] Robitaille and colleagues[59] showed that the GlideScope provided a better glottic view but did not significantly decrease movement of the nonpathologic cervical spine compared with DL. More recently, Kill and colleagues[60] found that GlideScope video-laryngoscopy reduced movements of the neck in patients with unsecured cervical spines, although the magnitude of differences were small, about 3°, and video motion analysis was used rather than fluoroscopy. Maruyama and colleagues[61] compared the AirWay scope with Macintosh blade DL with MILS and found that the AirWay scope decreased the median upper cervical spine movement during intubation in healthy volunteers. Turkstra and colleagues[57] found that the GlideScope resulted in reduced C2-C5 motion compared with DL in healthy volunteers. A recent comparison of the GlideScope and the C-MAC in immobilized patients found that tracheal intubation was more often successful on the first attempt with the GlideScope, and the C-MAC required significantly more optimizing maneuvers for success.[62] The influence on cervical spine motion was not assessed.

One crossover study in 23 volunteers compared success rates with awake Glide-Scope intubation and awake fiberoptic intubation after local anesthesia of the airway. The investigators found a 96% success rate with the GlideScope and 100% with fiber-optic intubation. The time to intubation was significant reduced in the GlideScope group. The investigators proposed that, among providers uncomfortable with flexible fiberoptic laryngoscopes, awake videolaryngoscopy was a feasible technique.[63] The benefit of this technique in patients with potential cervical spine instability is the allow-ance for a postintubation neurologic examination. However, with MILS, awake video-laryngoscopy may be prohibitively challenging.

In summary, videolaryngoscopy results in equivalent, possibly reduced cervical motion as DL, but may provide a better glottic view, which could be beneficial in immo-bilized patients with difficult airways requiring emergent intubation.

Lighted Optical Stylets

The light wand and other intubating stylets have also been studied in the context of cervical spine motion. Turkstra and colleagues[57] compared the light wand and DL in healthy volunteers intubated with MILS and showed reduced motion across all seg-ments with the light wand. Another study compared a lighted optical stylet with flexible fiberoptic bronchoscopic intubation and found no difference in the segmental cervical spine motion, but decreased time to intubation.[64] Recent comparisons of multiple airway devices in cadavers with experimental C5-C6 or C1-C2 ligamentous instability have shown significantly reduced motion in multiple planes with the light wand, compared with DL with MILS.[65,66] These studies did not show a difference in the time to intubation or incidence of failure with the light wand. Despite the reassuring evidence, the light wand may not be an appropriate first-line technique in patients with difficult airways, or for inexperienced operators, because it is a blind technique. The Shikani optical stylet provides the benefits of a lighted stylet and an indirect view of the vocal cords. Compared with DL, the Shikani was associated with significantly decreased cervical motion at all segments analyzed, but an increased risk of proce-dure failure.[67]

Supraglottic Airway Devices

Supraglottic airway devices are potentially dangerous for use in patients with unstable cervical spine disorders. Two recent studies documented high degrees of C1-C2 and

C4-C5 motion with the insertion of an intubating laryngeal mask airway (LMA) in cadavers with experimental cervical spine instability (about as much as DL).[65,66] Another study in patients undergoing cervical spine surgery found no difference in cervical flexion with the LMA compared with DL, but that the LMA produced motion in the opposite direction to DL.[68] The pressures exerted against the cervical vertebrae by intubating and classic LMAs have also been quantified as significantly increased compared with an endotracheal tube, and enough to produce posterior displacement of the cervical spine.[69] Ligamentous injuries have also been associated with LMA insertion in patients with unidentified cervical spine instability.[70] One recent study also documented a high rate of failure for blind intubation through an LMA in patients with neck immobilization.[71] Based on this information, the LMA should be reserved for cannot-intubate, cannot-ventilate scenarios.

Awake Flexible Fiberoptic Intubation

Awake fiberoptic intubation is the preferred technique in hemodynamically stable, cooperative patients with potentially unstable cervical spines.[52,72,73] Compared with rigid video laryngoscopy, flexible fiberoptic intubation was associated with significantly reduced cervical motion for every cervical motion angle analyzed.[74] Brimacombe and colleagues[75] found nasal fiberoptic intubation to result in less cervical motion to destabilized cadavers than a supraglottic airway, DL, intubating LMA, and mask ventilation. The drawbacks of fiberoptic intubation are that it requires the availability of advanced equipment, necessitates significant patient cooperation, and may be difficult for inexperienced providers to perform. Anxiolysis and sedation may not be feasible in otherwise unstable patients. In addition, time to intubation is significantly prolonged compared with other techniques.[64,76]

Future Studies

The existing studies that guide clinical decision making have primarily been conducted on human volunteers and by experimental manipulation of the cervical spine in human cadavers. Degrees of cervical motion or magnitudes of force measured in an unstable model are often unclearly translatable to clinical practice in a heterogeneous injured/at-risk population. However, randomized trials on patients with unstable cervical spine disorders are difficult to justify and subject to inadequate statistical power. The experimental evidence on human cadavers or healthy volunteers may be the best available evidence for the foreseeable future. Clinicians must carefully weigh the risks and benefits of each technique for airway management, and choose the one most likely to be successful on the first attempt. MILS should be performed with every intubation when cervical spine instability is suspected.

Extubation Failure and the Role of Tracheostomy

Careful extubation of the patient after cervical spine surgery is often underemphasized. Airway management that may have been difficult because of immobilization could be even more challenging after spinal fusion. Prolonged prone positioning can result in upper airway edema, and postoperative hematoma formation may result in airway compromise. A recent series of 311 patients after cervical spine surgery found a rate of airway complications of 6.1%.[77] Predictors of airway complications were involvement of more than 3 vertebral levels, blood loss greater than 300 mL, upper cervical vertebral instrumentation, operative time greater than 5 hours, and combined anterior-posterior approach.[78] Presence of 1 or more of the these factors may warrant delayed extubation.

In patients with severe cervical spinal cord injury, respiratory muscle weakness may also be present and predispose patients to prolonged need for mechanical ventilation.[79] A recent observational study of patients with cervical spinal cord injury measured a tracheostomy rate of 10%.[80] Predictors for tracheostomy in this series included age more than 69 years, severe neurologic impairment score, low forced vital capacity (<500 mL), and low percentage of actual to predicted vital capacity. These data and others suggest that early tracheostomy may be warranted in patients with high injury/impairment scores.[81,82] Early tracheostomy has also been associated with decreased hospital length of stay, earlier phonation, earlier decannulation, and decreased hospital costs.[83]

SUMMARY

Airway management of patients with cervical spinal cord instability involves many variables and potentially predisposes patients to secondary neurologic injury. Spinal cord instability is most common in patients with trauma; however, there are several congenital and acquired conditions that predispose the cervical spine to instability. Patterns of injury/instability are often heterogeneous and, even though the risk of neurologic complications is low, the cost is extremely high. For this reason, every patient with suspected instability should receive immobilization during airway management with MILS. The selection of airway management technique depends on individual patient factors such as characteristics of injury, risk of aspiration and hypoxia, clinician experience, and patient cooperation. From the existing observational data, it seems that the best strategy for airway management is one that applies the technique with both the highest likelihood of success on the first attempt and the lowest biomechanical influence on a potentially unstable spine.

REFERENCES

1. Benzel EC, Waxman SG, Byrne TN. Diseases of the spine and spinal cord. Cary (NC): Oxford University Press; 2000.
2. White AA 3rd, Johnson RM, Panjabi MM, et al. Biomechanical analysis of clinical stability in the cervical spine. Clin Orthop Relat Res 1975;(109):85–96.
3. Singh A, Tetreault L, Kalsi-Ryan S, et al. Global prevalence and incidence of traumatic spinal cord injury. Clin Epidemiol 2014;6:309–31.
4. Hasler RM, Exadaktylos AK, Bouamra O, et al. Epidemiology and predictors of cervical spine injury in adult major trauma patients: a multicenter cohort study. J Trauma Acute Care Surg 2012;72(4):975–81.
5. Demetriades D, Charalambides K, Chahwan S, et al. Nonskeletal cervical spine injuries: Epidemiology and diagnostic pitfalls. J Trauma 2000;48(4):724–7.
6. Holly LT, Kelly DF, Counelis GJ, et al. Cervical spine trauma associated with moderate and severe head injury: incidence, risk factors, and injury characteristics. J Neurosurg 2002;96(3 Suppl):285–91.
7. Hackl W, Hausberger K, Sailer R, et al. Prevalence of cervical spine injuries in patients with facial trauma. Oral Surg Oral Med Oral Pathol Oral Radiol Endod 2001;92(4):370–6.
8. Goldberg W, Mueller C, Panacek E, et al. Distribution and patterns of blunt traumatic cervical spine injury. Ann Emerg Med 2001;38(1):17–21.
9. Karbi OA, Caspari DA, Tator CH. Extrication, immobilization and radiologic investigation of patients with cervical spine injuries. CMAJ 1988;139(7):617–21.
10. Chapman J, Smith JS, Kopjar B, et al. The AOSpine North America Geriatric Odontoid Fracture Mortality Study: a retrospective review of mortality outcomes

for operative versus nonoperative treatment of 322 patients with long-term follow-up. Spine (Phila Pa 1976) 2013;38(13):1098–104.

11. Cha TD, An HS. Cervical spine manifestations in patients with inflammatory arthritides. Nat Rev Rheumatol 2013;9(7):423–32.

12. Joaquim AF, Appenzeller S. Cervical spine involvement in rheumatoid arthritis — A systematic review. Autoimmun Rev 2014;13(12):1195–202.

13. Broom MJ, Raycroft JF. Complications of fractures of the cervical spine in ankylosing spondylitis. Spine (Phila Pa 1976) 1988;13(7):763–6.

14. Podolsky SM, Hoffman JR, Pietrafesa CA. Neurologic complications following immobilization of cervical spine fracture in a patient with ankylosing spondylitis. Ann Emerg Med 1983;12(9):578–80.

15. Caron T, Bransford R, Nguyen Q, et al. Spine fractures in patients with ankylosing spinal disorders. Spine (Phila Pa 1976) 2010;35(11):E458–64.

16. McKay SD, Al-Omari A, Tomlinson LA, et al. Review of cervical spine anomalies in genetic syndromes. Spine (Phila Pa 1976) 2012;37(5):E269–77.

17. Hoffman JR, Mower WR, Wolfson AB, et al. Validity of a set of clinical criteria to rule out injury to the cervical spine in patients with blunt trauma. National emergency X-radiography utilization study group. N Engl J Med 2000;343(2):94–9.

18. Stiell IG, Wells GA, Vandemheen KL, et al. The Canadian C-spine rule for radiography in alert and stable trauma patients. JAMA 2001;286(15):1841–8.

19. Michaleff ZA, Maher CG, Verhagen AP, et al. Accuracy of the Canadian C-spine rule and NEXUS to screen for clinically important cervical spine injury in patients following blunt trauma: a systematic review. CMAJ 2012;184(16):E867–76.

20. Stiell IG, Clement CM, McKnight RD, et al. The Canadian C-spine rule versus the NEXUS low-risk criteria in patients with trauma. N Engl J Med 2003;349(26):2510–8.

21. Schenarts PJ, Diaz J, Kaiser C, et al. Prospective comparison of admission computed tomographic scan and plain films of the upper cervical spine in trauma patients with altered mental status. J Trauma 2001;51(4):663–8 [discussion: 668–9].

22. Brohi K, Healy M, Fotheringham T, et al. Helical computed tomographic scanning for the evaluation of the cervical spine in the unconscious, intubated trauma patient. J Trauma 2005;58(5):897–901.

23. Stassen NA, Williams VA, Gestring ML, et al. Magnetic resonance imaging in combination with helical computed tomography provides a safe and efficient method of cervical spine clearance in the obtunded trauma patient. J Trauma 2006;60(1):171–7.

24. Morris CG, McCoy E. Clearing the cervical spine in unconscious polytrauma victims, balancing risks and effective screening. Anaesthesia 2004;59(5):464–82.

25. D'Alise MD, Benzel EC, Hart BL. Magnetic resonance imaging evaluation of the cervical spine in the comatose or obtunded trauma patient. J Neurosurg 1999;91(1 Suppl):54–9.

26. Benzel EC, Hart BL, Ball PA, et al. Magnetic resonance imaging for the evaluation of patients with occult cervical spine injury. J Neurosurg 1996;85(5):824–9.

27. Domeier RM, Swor RA, Evans RW, et al. Multicenter prospective validation of prehospital clinical spinal clearance criteria. J Trauma 2002;53(4):744–50.

28. Cervical spine immobilization before admission to the hospital. Neurosurgery 2002;50(3 Suppl):S7–17.

29. Podolsky S, Baraff LJ, Simon RR, et al. Efficacy of cervical spine immobilization methods. J Trauma 1983;23(6):461–5.

30. Goutcher CM, Lochhead V. Reduction in mouth opening with semi-rigid cervical collars. Br J Anaesth 2005;95(3):344–8.

31. Aprahamian C, Thompson BM, Finger WA, et al. Experimental cervical spine injury model: Evaluation of airway management and splinting techniques. Ann Emerg Med 1984;13(8):584–7.
32. Hauswald M, Sklar DP, Tandberg D, et al. Cervical spine movement during airway management: Cinefluoroscopic appraisal in human cadavers. Am J Emerg Med 1991;9(6):535–8.
33. Donaldson WF 3rd, Heil BV, Donaldson VP, et al. The effect of airway maneuvers on the unstable C1-C2 segment. A cadaver study. Spine (Phila Pa 1976) 1997; 22(11):1215–8.
34. Helliwell V, Gabbott DA. The effect of single-handed cricoid pressure on cervical spine movement after applying manual in-line stabilisation – a cadaver study. Resuscitation 2001;49(1):53–7.
35. Aoi Y, Inagawa G, Hashimoto K, et al. Airway scope laryngoscopy under manual inline stabilization and cervical collar immobilization: a crossover in vivo cine-fluoroscopic study. J Trauma 2011;71(1):32–6.
36. Manoach S, Paladino L. Manual in-line stabilization for acute airway management of suspected cervical spine injury: historical review and current questions. Ann Emerg Med 2007;50(3):236–45.
37. Kwan I, Bunn F, Roberts I. Spinal immobilisation for trauma patients. Cochrane Database Syst Rev 2001;(2):CD002803.
38. Farmer J, Vaccaro A, Albert TJ, et al. Neurologic deterioration after cervical spinal cord injury. J Spinal Disord 1998;11(3):192–6.
39. McLeod AD, Calder I. Spinal cord injury and direct laryngoscopy–the legend lives on. Br J Anaesth 2000;84(6):705–9.
40. Muckart DJ, Bhagwanjee S, van der Merwe R. Spinal cord injury as a result of endotracheal intubation in patients with undiagnosed cervical spine fractures. Anesthesiology 1997;87(2):418–20.
41. Hastings RH, Wood PR. Head extension and laryngeal view during laryngoscopy with cervical spine stabilization maneuvers. Anesthesiology 1994;80(4): 825–31.
42. Gerling MC, Davis DP, Hamilton RS, et al. Effects of cervical spine immobilization technique and laryngoscope blade selection on an unstable cervical spine in a cadaver model of intubation. Ann Emerg Med 2000;36(4):293–300.
43. Lennarson PJ, Smith DW, Sawin PD, et al. Cervical spinal motion during intubation: Efficacy of stabilization maneuvers in the setting of complete segmental instability. J Neurosurg 2001;94(2 Suppl):265–70.
44. Lennarson PJ, Smith D, Todd MM, et al. Segmental cervical spine motion during orotracheal intubation of the intact and injured spine with and without external stabilization. J Neurosurg 2000;92(2 Suppl):201–6.
45. Nolan JP, Wilson ME. Orotracheal intubation in patients with potential cervical spine injuries. An indication for the gum elastic bougie. Anaesthesia 1993; 48(7):630–3.
46. Grande CM, Barton CR, Stene JK. Appropriate techniques for airway management of emergency patients with suspected spinal cord injury. Anesth Analg 1988;67(7):714–5.
47. Stephens CT, Kahntroff S, Dutton RP. The success of emergency endotracheal intubation in trauma patients: a 10-year experience at a major adult trauma referral center. Anesth Analg 2009;109(3):866–72.
48. Sawin PD, Todd MM, Traynelis VC, et al. Cervical spine motion with direct laryngoscopy and orotracheal intubation. An in vivo cinefluoroscopic study of subjects without cervical abnormality. Anesthesiology 1996;85(1):26–36.

49. LeGrand SA, Hindman BJ, Dexter F, et al. Craniocervical motion during direct laryngoscopy and orotracheal intubation with the Macintosh and Miller blades: an in vivo cinefluoroscopic study. Anesthesiology 2007;107(6):884–91.
50. Crosby ET. Airway management in adults after cervical spine trauma. Anesthesiology 2006;104(6):1293–318.
51. Shatney CH, Brunner RD, Nguyen TQ. The safety of orotracheal intubation in patients with unstable cervical spine fracture or high spinal cord injury. Am J Surg 1995;170(6):676–9 [discussion: 679–80].
52. Lord SA, Boswell WC, Williams JS, et al. Airway control in trauma patients with cervical spine fractures. Prehosp Disaster Med 1994;9(1):44–9.
53. Aziz M. Airway management in neuroanesthesiology. Anesthesiol Clin 2012;30(2): 229–40.
54. Aziz M. Use of video-assisted intubation devices in the management of patients with trauma. Anesthesiol Clin 2013;31(1):157–66.
55. Malik MA, Maharaj CH, Harte BH, et al. Comparison of Macintosh, Truview EVO2, Glidescope, and Airwayscope laryngoscope use in patients with cervical spine immobilization. Br J Anaesth 2008;101(5):723–30.
56. Wetsch WA, Spelten O, Hellmich M, et al. Comparison of different video laryngoscopes for emergency intubation in a standardized airway manikin with immobilized cervical spine by experienced anaesthetists. A randomized, controlled crossover trial. Resuscitation 2012;83(6):740–5.
57. Turkstra TP, Craen RA, Pelz DM, et al. Cervical spine motion: a fluoroscopic comparison during intubation with lighted stylet, GlideScope, and Macintosh laryngoscope. Anesth Analg 2005;101(3):910–5 Table of contents.
58. Hindman BJ, Santoni BG, Puttlitz CM, et al. Intubation biomechanics: laryngoscope force and cervical spine motion during intubation with Macintosh and Airtraq laryngoscopes. Anesthesiology 2014;121(2):260–71.
59. Robitaille A, Williams SR, Tremblay MH, et al. Cervical spine motion during tracheal intubation with manual in-line stabilization: direct laryngoscopy versus GlideScope videolaryngoscopy. Anesth Analg 2008;106(3):935–41 Table of contents.
60. Kill C, Risse J, Wallot P, et al. Videolaryngoscopy with Glidescope reduces cervical spine movement in patients with unsecured cervical spine. J Emerg Med 2013;44(4):750–6.
61. Maruyama K, Yamada T, Kawakami R, et al. Randomized cross-over comparison of cervical-spine motion with the AirWay scope or Macintosh laryngoscope with in-line stabilization: a video-fluoroscopic study. Br J Anaesth 2008;101(4):563–7.
62. Bruck S, Trautner H, Wolff A, et al. Comparison of the C-MAC and GlideScope videolaryngoscopes in patients with cervical spine disorders and immobilisation. Anaesthesia 2015;70(2):160–5.
63. Silverton NA, Youngquist ST, Mallin MP, et al. GlideScope versus flexible fiber optic for awake upright laryngoscopy. Ann Emerg Med 2012;59(3):159–64.
64. Houde BJ, Williams SR, Cadrin-Chenevert A, et al. A comparison of cervical spine motion during orotracheal intubation with the Trachlight® or the flexible fiberoptic bronchoscope. Anesth Analg 2009;108(5):1638–43.
65. Prasarn ML, Conrad B, Rubery PT, et al. Comparison of 4 airway devices on cervical spine alignment in a cadaver model with global ligamentous instability at C5-C6. Spine (Phila Pa 1976) 2012;37(6):476–81.
66. Wendling AL, Tighe PJ, Conrad BP, et al. A comparison of 4 airway devices on cervical spine alignment in cadaver models of global ligamentous instability at C1-2. Anesth Analg 2013;117(1):126–32.

67. Turkstra TP, Pelz DM, Shaikh AA, et al. Cervical spine motion: a fluoroscopic comparison of Shikani Optical Stylet vs Macintosh laryngoscope. Can J Anaesth 2007;54(6):441–7.

68. Kihara S, Watanabe S, Brimacombe J, et al. Segmental cervical spine movement with the intubating laryngeal mask during manual in-line stabilization in patients with cervical pathology undergoing cervical spine surgery. Anesth Analg 2000; 91(1):195–200.

69. Keller C, Brimacombe J, Keller K. Pressures exerted against the cervical vertebrae by the standard and intubating laryngeal mask airways: a randomized, controlled, cross-over study in fresh cadavers. Anesth Analg 1999;89(5): 1296–300.

70. Edge CJ, Hyman N, Addy V, et al. Posterior spinal ligament rupture associated with laryngeal mask insertion in a patient with undisclosed unstable cervical spine. Br J Anaesth 2002;89(3):514–7.

71. Wakeling HG, Nightingale J. The intubating laryngeal mask airway does not facilitate tracheal intubation in the presence of a neck collar in simulated trauma. Br J Anaesth 2000;84(2):254–6.

72. Fuchs G, Schwarz G, Baumgartner A, et al. Fiberoptic intubation in 327 neurosurgical patients with lesions of the cervical spine. J Neurosurg Anesthesiol 1999; 11(1):11–6.

73. Manninen PH, Jose GB, Lukitto K, et al. Management of the airway in patients undergoing cervical spine surgery. J Neurosurg Anesthesiol 2007;19(3):190–4.

74. Wong DM, Prabhu A, Chakraborty S, et al. Cervical spine motion during flexible bronchoscopy compared with the lo-pro GlideScope. Br J Anaesth 2009;102(3): 424–30.

75. Brimacombe J, Keller C, Kunzel KH, et al. Cervical spine motion during airway management: a cinefluoroscopic study of the posteriorly destabilized third cervical vertebrae in human cadavers. Anesth Analg 2000;91(5):1274–8.

76. Cohn AI, Zornow MH. Awake endotracheal intubation in patients with cervical spine disease: a comparison of the Bullard laryngoscope and the fiberoptic bronchoscope. Anesth Analg 1995;81(6):1283–6.

77. Sagi HC, Beutler W, Carroll E, et al. Airway complications associated with surgery on the anterior cervical spine. Spine (Phila Pa 1976) 2002;27(9):949–53.

78. Terao Y, Matsumoto S, Yamashita K, et al. Increased incidence of emergency airway management after combined anterior-posterior cervical spine surgery. J Neurosurg Anesthesiol 2004;16(4):282–6.

79. Kornblith LZ, Kutcher ME, Callcut RA, et al. Mechanical ventilation weaning and extubation after spinal cord injury: a western trauma association multicenter study. J Trauma Acute Care Surg 2013;75(6):1060–9 [discussion: 1069–70].

80. Yugue I, Okada S, Ueta T, et al. Analysis of the risk factors for tracheostomy in traumatic cervical spinal cord injury. Spine (Phila Pa 1976) 2012;37(26):E1633–8.

81. Menaker J, Kufera JA, Glaser J, et al. Admission ASIA motor score predicting the need for tracheostomy after cervical spinal cord injury. J Trauma Acute Care Surg 2013;75(4):629–34.

82. Como JJ, Sutton ER, McCunn M, et al. Characterizing the need for mechanical ventilation following cervical spinal cord injury with neurologic deficit. J Trauma 2005;59(4):912–6 [discussion: 916].

83. Cameron TS, McKinstry A, Burt SK, et al. Outcomes of patients with spinal cord injury before and after introduction of an interdisciplinary tracheostomy team. Crit Care Resusc 2009;11(1):14–9.

Infections and Edema

Gary Linkov, MD[a], Ahmed M.S. Soliman, MD[b],*

KEYWORDS

- Deep neck infection • Retropharyngeal abscess • Ludwig angina
- Peritonsillar abscess • Supraglottitis • Hereditary angioedema
- ACE inhibitor angioedema • Allergic angioedema

KEY POINTS

- Infection and angioedema of the head and neck are common causes of impaired airways.
- History, physical examination, and fiberoptic laryngoscopy are critical in evaluation.
- Preintervention discussion and planning by anesthesia and otolaryngology are essential.
- A decision regarding the primary modality and contingency plans to secure the airway is made.
- Regular practice by the entire team in simulation laboratories will maintain and hone skills.

INTRODUCTION

Infectious and inflammatory conditions of the head and neck often present with impaired and challenging airways. Careful evaluation and accurate diagnosis will allow for prompt and safe management of the airway and the treatment of the underlying condition. Development of primary and contingency plans for securing the airway is critical and requires discussion and coordination between the anesthesiologist and otolaryngologist. This article focuses on the evaluation and management of patients with infections involving the upper aerodigestive tract and neck as well as angioedema.

DEEP NECK INFECTIONS

The occurrence of deep neck infections has been declining since the introduction of antibiotics. Deep neck infections are generally polymicrobial. *Streptococci*, *Peptostreptococcus*, *Staphylococcus*, and anaerobes are the organisms most commonly cultured. These bacteria are generally part of the normal oral flora but become virulent when mucosal barriers are violated.[1]

[a] Temple University Hospital, Philadelphia, PA 19140, USA; [b] Department of Otolaryngology-Head & Neck Surgery, Voice, Airway & Swallowing Center, Temple University School of Medicine, 3440 North Broad Street Kresge West 312, Philadelphia, PA 19140, USA
* Corresponding author.
E-mail address: asoliman@temple.edu

Anesthesiology Clin 33 (2015) 329–346
http://dx.doi.org/10.1016/j.anclin.2015.02.005
1932-2275/15/$ – see front matter © 2015 Elsevier Inc. All rights reserved.

anesthesiology.theclinics.com

Successful management of deep neck infections often involves control of the airway, effective antibiotic therapy, and timely surgical intervention. A focused history and physical examination should be obtained if possible, followed by either control of the airway if compromised, imaging to assess extent of infection, and surgical drainage if needed. Patients may present with generalized symptoms of fever and malaise or with more localizing symptoms of shortness of breath, odynophagia, dysphagia, sore throat, neck pain, stiffness, or voice changes. The most common finding on examination is neck swelling.[2,3] The examiner may also note dyspnea, stridor, elevation, or firmness in the floor of the mouth, fever, and pharyngeal wall or soft palate swelling. Although rare, bleeding may be related to a sentinel bleed from infectious involvement of the carotid artery. Tachypnea or stridor may indicate impending airway obstruction and mandate immediate attention.[4]

The parapharyngeal (lateral pharyngeal) space is the most commonly involved space (38.4%) in several large studies.[5] Odontogenic and upper airway infections are the 2 most common causes of deep neck infections (53% and 31%, respectively).[1,6] Streptococcus viridans and Klebsiella pneumoniae were the most common organisms (34% each). In another large retrospective review of 234 patients, deep neck infections were the first manifestation of a malignant tumor in 6% of cases, which should raise awareness that an infected tumor may present as a deep neck space infection.[7]

Submandibular Space

Submandibular space infections can involve either of the 2 subcompartments, the sublingual or the submylohyoid, or both. These 2 subcompartments communicate posteriorly around the mylohyoid muscle. Ludwig angina is the name for the prototypical infection of the submandibular space infection and requires that both compartments be involved. An odontogenic source of infection is identified in 70% to 85% of cases. Other causes may include a floor-of-mouth laceration, mandibular trauma, tumor, sialadenitis, or lymphadenitis. The most frequent bacterial isolate is the α-hemolytic Streptococcus. The distensible tissue in the floor of the mouth can be pushed superiorly, displacing the tongue posteriorly, and decreasing its range of motion (Fig. 1A). On examination, the suprahyoid neck is often tender with woody induration with rare fluctuance (see Fig. 1B). Computed tomography (CT) may show a collection (Fig. 2). Infection may spread from the submandibular space to the lateral pharyngeal space by way of the buccopharyngeal gap created by the styloglossus muscle, further complicating the situation.[4]

Airway management in this group can be quite challenging. Standard direct laryngoscopy with a Mac or Miller blade will often fail because of the floor-of-mouth firmness and retro-displacement of the tongue. Awake nasal fiberoptic intubation is usually the best option, with the patient sitting up and their head in the sniffing position. This position maximally opens the pharyngeal airway to allow for passage of the endotracheal tube (ETT). It allows assessment of the airway, which is helpful in planning for extubation. Wire-reinforced anode ETT are ideal for this purpose because of their flexibility; smaller sizes[6,7] are used because their outer diameter is slightly larger than the standard polyvinyl chloride ETTs. The nostrils are first decongested and anesthetized with a mixture of 0.05% oxymetazoline and 4% lidocaine on 1/2 × 3-inch Cottonoids followed by dilation using soft silicone nasal airways lubricated with 4% lidocaine jelly (Figs. 3–6). Pretreatment with intravenous dexmedetomidine makes this process considerably easier because it allows for sedation without significant suppression of the respiratory drive. Oxygen is usually delivered via a nasal cannula placed between the teeth during the intubation. The otolaryngologist should be prepared for tracheotomy if fiberoptic intubation is not successful (Boxes 1 and 2, Table 1).

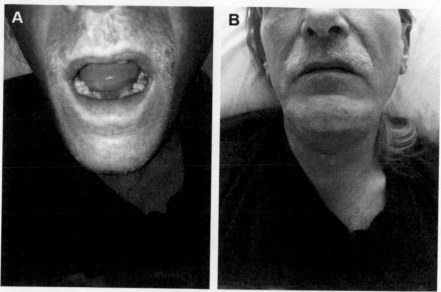

Fig. 1. (*A*) Submandibular space abscess with superior extension into sublingual space posteriorly displacing the tongue. (*B*) Submandibular space abscess with suprahyoid induration and swelling.

Alternatively, awake tracheotomy may be used as the primary method for securing the airway and may be preferred when there is significant narrowing of the oropharyngeal airway or significant edema of the floor of the mouth. In this subset of patients, there may be a need for prolonged airway protection while the edema subsides. In

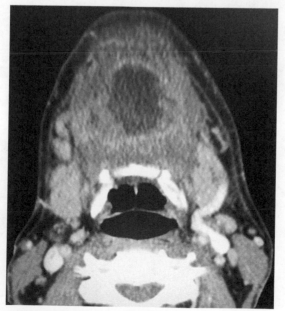

Fig. 2. Axial CT showing submandibular fluid collection.

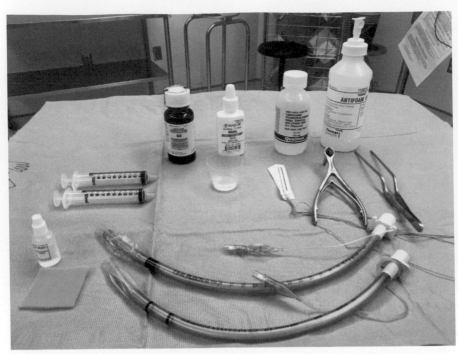

Fig. 3. Setup for awake nasal fiberoptic intubation.

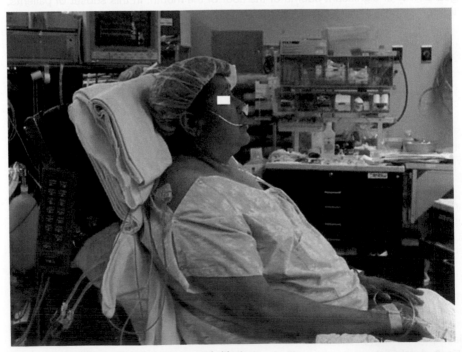

Fig. 4. Awake fiberoptic intubation-nasal dilation.

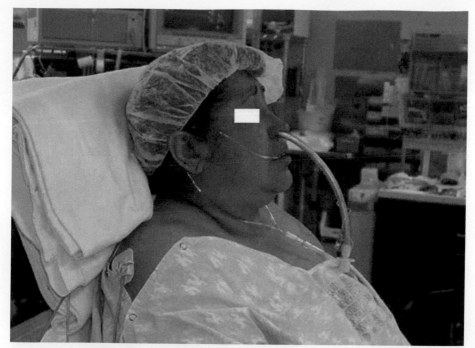

Fig. 5. Awake fiberoptic intubation-nasal placement of ETT.

the absence of in-hospital personnel with experience in difficult airway management, tracheotomy provides a more secure airway and a safer postoperative course. Elevating the patient's back approximately 30° and using a small shoulder roll to extend the neck will allow them to breathe comfortably while providing adequate access to the neck (**Fig. 7**). Great care needs to be taken to ensure that oxygen is not delivered while electrocautery is being used because of the fire risk. The harmonic scalpel may be useful in this situation because it functions via mechanical vibration rather than electrical current and does not cause sparking on the surgical field.

High-dose intravenous penicillin and clindamycin are the antibiotics of choice. Surgical drainage can be intraoral or via external incision. Intraoral drainage is reserved for uncomplicated submandibular space infections limited to the sublingual compartment; otherwise, an external approach is warranted. The external incision is made only after the airway has been adequately controlled (**Fig. 8**).[4]

The safety of extubation after surgery is determined by the preoperative examination, extent of infection, and adequacy of surgical drainage. In cases of extensive preoperative airway edema or where tissue induration and edema is identified rather than a large collection of pus, extubation may be imprudent. Tracheotomy should be considered in these cases.

Lateral Pharyngeal Space

Infection can enter the lateral pharyngeal (parapharyngeal space) space via lateral extension from the peritonsillar space, posterior extension from the submandibular space, anterior extension from retropharyngeal space, or medial extension from the deep parotid space. The lateral pharyngeal space is separated from the peritonsillar space by the superior constrictor muscle. The anterior compartment (prestyloid) of

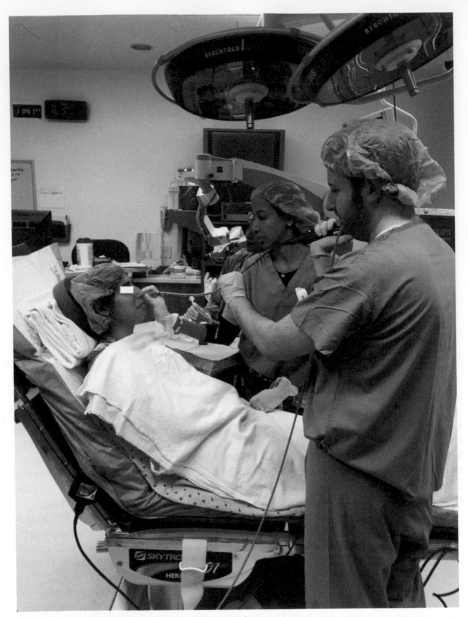

Fig. 6. Awake fiberoptic intubation-fiberoptic laryngoscopy.

the lateral pharyngeal space contains fat, connective tissue, lymph nodes, and muscle, whereas the posterior compartment (poststyloid) contains the carotid sheath and cranial nerves IX, X, XII. Infections typically present about 1 week after a tonsillitis or pharyngitis. Clinical signs may include trismus (indicating that the pterygoid musculature is involved), swelling near the angle of mandible, medial bulging of the lateral pharyngeal wall, or systemic toxicity.[4]

Because the carotid sheath lies within the posterior compartment of the lateral pharyngeal space, vascular complications may arise from aggressive or untreated

Box 1
Epiglottitis protocol

I. Once the diagnosis of epiglottitis is suspected, the following steps are to be followed without exception:

  A. Begin continuous observation of the patient.

    Allow the parents to remain with the patient.

    Do not place the child in a supine position.

  B. Contact the team designated to secure the airway: anesthesiologist, intensivist, otolaryngologist.

  C. Place equipment for bag/face mask ventilation, intubation, oxygen, suction, tracheostomy, and cardiopulmonary resuscitation at bedside.

  D. Do not agitate the child with noxious procedures such as oral examination, blood drawing, or intravenous (IV) catheter placement.

  E. Begin continuous electrocardiogram, respiratory, and pulse oximetry monitoring.

  F. Obtain lateral neck roentgenogram only if the child is stable and the diagnosis is uncertain.

    A physician capable of intubation must accompany the child to the radiology department.

  G. Administer oxygen at 1 to 2 L/min or at a rate sufficient to maintain oxygen saturation greater than 90% by pulse oximetry.

  H. Consider administering nebulized racemic epinephrine (2.25%) at 0.2 mL in 2 mL 0.9% sodium chloride solution for worsening airway obstruction.

  I. If complete airway obstruction occurs before the arrival of the airway team, begin assisted ventilation with bag and face mask.

II. Once the airway team has arrived, perform the following:

  A. Transport the child to the operating room or pediatric intensive care unit (PICU).

  B. Ask the otolaryngologist to be prepared for fiberoptic examination, rigid bronchoscopy, or tracheostomy and to remain in the room.

  C. Induce anesthesia with the patient in a sitting position using an inhalation agent and oxygen.

    Confirm the diagnosis of epiglottitis.

    Intubate the child through the oral route with an ETT one size smaller than recommended for that age patient.

  D. Hyperoxygenate the child for 2 minutes.

    Replace the oral ETT with a nasotracheal tube.

  E. Obtain a chest roentgenogram to ensure proper placement of the ETT and to evaluate for pulmonary abnormalities.

  F. Place an IV catheter; obtain blood and pharyngeal cultures.

  G. Begin antibiotic therapy.

  H. Transfer to the PICU after administering a sedative (eg, midazolam) and placing arm restraints.

From Al-Sundi S. Acute upper airway obstruction: croup, epiglottitis, bacterial tracheitis, and retropharyngeal abrasions. In: Levin D, Morris F, editors. Essentials of pediatric intensive care. New York: Churchill Livingstone; 1997; with permission.

Box 2
Checklist for awake fiberoptic intubation

Bayonette forceps

Nasal speculum

$1/2 \times$ 3-inch nasal pledgets

4% lidocaine

0.05% oxymetazoline

Lidocaine jelly

Lubricant spray for bronchoscope

Antifog drops for bronchoscope

10-cc syringe with slip tip ×2

Nasal airway 16–32 Fr

Wire reinforced (anode) ETTs 6, 6.5, 7, 7.5 mm

Flexible bronchoscope

---

infections in this area. The most common of these is a suppurative internal jugular vein thrombosis, which can potentially lead to bacteremia, septic pulmonary emboli, lateral and cavernous sinus thrombosis, or metastatic abscess formation. The most feared vascular complication is carotid artery erosion, which most commonly affects the internal carotid artery and may be heralded by smaller sentinel bleeds from the mouth, nose, or ear.

As in submandibular space infections, the 3 central tenets of therapy are airway control, antimicrobials, and surgical drainage. Flexible laryngoscopy is extremely useful in assessing the airway before any intervention. In cases with adequate mouth opening and limited medial encroachment by the abscess, standard direct laryngoscopy with a Mac or Miller blade and orotracheal intubation is often successful. Use of the Glide Scope allows the anesthesia and otolaryngology teams to both visualize the

---

Table 1
Airway management plan with contingencies for various pathologies

Airway Obstruction	A	B	C
DNI: Submandibular	NF	AT	—
DNI: Lateral pharyngeal wall	OI	NF	AT
DNI: Retropharyngeal	OI	NF	AT
UA: Tonsillitis/PTA	OI	NF	AT
UA: Supraglottitis	NF	AT	—
AE: Tongue	NF	AT	—
AE: Larynx	NF	AT	—

Cause of airway obstruction and preferred strategies to secure airway: "A" denotes the first strategy to try if clinical presentation permits. Of note, depending on the severity of presenting signs and symptoms, the above data will need to be tailored to the individual patient. More than one methodology may be appropriate.

Abbreviations: AE, angioedema; AT, awake tracheotomy; DNI, deep neck infection; NF, nasal fiberoptic; OI, oral intubation; PTA, peritonsillar abscess; UA, upper airway.

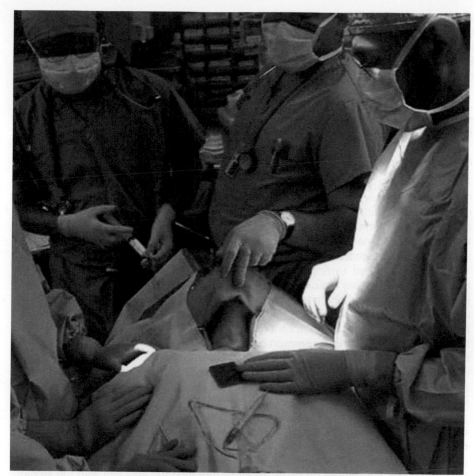

Fig. 7. Positioning of patient for awake tracheotomy.

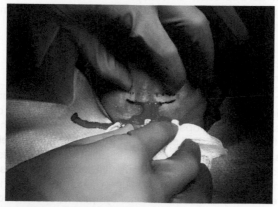

Fig. 8. Submandibular space abscess drained.

anatomy and allay much of the associated anxiety. Awake nasal fiberoptic intubation using the contralateral nostril is often the preferred technique when significant trismus is present; however, there needs to be adequate space in the oropharynx to pass the ETT. If there is significant obstruction of the pharyngeal airway, awake tracheotomy may be required.

The preferred access to the lateral pharyngeal space is via an external approach, using a lateral submandibular incision with dissection medial to the angle of the mandible to enter the lateral pharyngeal space.[4] Anaerobes play a greater role in this space, generally requiring treatment with either clindamycin or metronidazole.

Retropharyngeal Space

The retropharyngeal space involves 2 chains of lymphatics that lie just off of the midline and usually involute by age 5, which explains the rarity of these infections in older patients. Sources of infection in this location include trauma, instrumentation, endotracheal intubation, placement of a nasogastric tube, and spread of infection from other deep neck spaces. When the infection is caudal to the nasopharynx, swelling of the posterior pharyngeal wall will be seen just off midline on examination. Additional signs and symptoms may include cervical adenopathy, irritability, and nuchal rigidity. Severe respiratory distress should raise suspicion for mediastinal extension. The retropharyngeal space communicates with the anterior and posterior aspects of the superior mediastinum, and consequently, potential complications include mediastinitis, pyopneumothorax, bronchial erosion, and purulent pericarditis.[4] Mediastinitis was the most common complication noted (6%) in a large retrospective review in 2012.[1] When these life-threatening complications occur, the mortality increases significantly and ranges from 7% to 42%. The only significant prognostic factor for the onset of complications based on a recent multivariate analysis was the involvement of more than one neck space.[3]

Treatment of retropharyngeal abscesses involves intravenous antibiotics and surgical drainage. Preoperative flexible laryngoscopy and review of the CT scan will determine the extent of anterior encroachment and guide airway management (**Fig. 9**). In uncomplicated cases, standard direct laryngoscopy and orotracheal intubation may be carried out. Care must be taken to avoid rupturing the abscess with the laryngoscope or ETT and to put the patient in a slight Trendelenburg position and have suction readily available if this were to happen. Large abscesses with significant airway narrowing are best managed with awake tracheotomy before drainage. Most of these will require an external approach[8] whereby an incision is made anterior to the sternocleidomastoid muscle. If there is mediastinal extension, the patient may require either thoracotomy or thoracoscopy to complete the drainage.

UPPER AERODIGESTIVE TRACT INFECTIONS
Pharyngotonsillar Infections

Pharyngotonsillar infections include pharyngitis, tonsillitis, and peritonsillar infections. Viruses, such as influenza and parainfluenza, are the most common cause of pharyngitis and tonsillitis in all age groups. Group A streptococci (GAS) is the most common bacterial cause of pharyngitis. The significance of GAS infection is related to its association with both suppurative complications, such as otitis media, sinusitis, and peritonsillar and deep neck infections, and nonsuppurative sequelae, such as acute rheumatic fever and glomerulonephritis. Symptoms suggestive of nonstrep pharyngitis include concurrent viral respiratory or gastrointestinal symptoms, such as cough, rhinorrhea, conjunctivitis, and diarrhea. Symptoms and signs of GAS include tonsillar exudates,

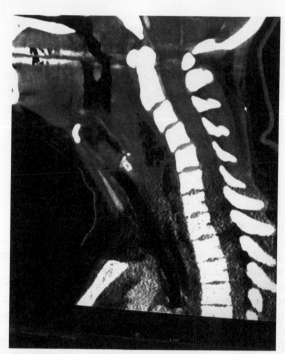

Fig. 9. Sagittal CT demonstrating retropharyngeal abscess.

swollen and tender cervical lymphadenopathy, lack of cough, and presence of fever. Penicillin-based antibiotics are the therapeutic drugs of choice.[9]

A peritonsillar abscess forms when the oral flora invades the peritonsillar space forming an abscess between the palatine tonsil and its capsule. The patient typically complains of a sore throat that is worse on one side, unilateral otalgia, fever, and trismus. On examination, classically the patient has pharyngeal erythema, asymmetric peritonsillar swelling, soft palate bulging with deviation of the uvula away from the side of infection, and limited mouth opening (**Fig. 10**). The presence of trismus is more likely to be associated with abscess rather than cellulitis or phlegmon.

Confirmation of a diagnosis can be made with needle aspiration, ultrasound, or CT (**Fig. 11**). Treatment is with either bedside aspiration or intraoral incision and drainage, followed by pain control and antibiotics. Intravenous steroids have also been shown to speed symptom resolution.[8] Airway compromise is very rare, with an isolated peritonsillar abscess, and may signify extension to adjacent deep neck spaces, including the retropharyngeal space or lateral pharyngeal space.[10]

Airway compromise is more likely with mononucleosis, which results in hypertrophy of the lymphoid tissue in Waldeyer ring, including the tonsils bilaterally, adenoids, and lingual tonsils. Patients are also usually more ill with fatigue and a more protracted course. This diagnosis may be made in many cases using a Monospot test and readily responds to corticosteroids.[11]

Supraglottitis

Supraglottitis, sometimes referred to as epiglottitis, is an inflammatory condition of the supraglottic larynx that can rapidly progress to life-threatening airway obstruction. Historically, supraglottitis was closely associated with *Haemophilus influenzae* type b (Hib) infection. Since the early 1990s, however, primarily due to the Hib vaccine,

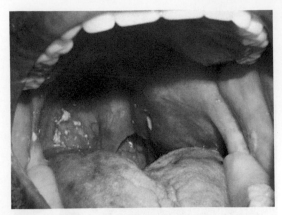

Fig. 10. Left peritonsillar abscess.

there has been a significant decline in the number of cases of childhood supraglottitis. Meanwhile, the incidence of supraglottitis in adults has risen.

Although Hib-related supraglottitis is still reported in both immunized and nonimmunized children, more commonly now *Streptococci* and *Staphylococci* organisms are the cause.[9] Of note, Shah and colleagues[12] reported on 6 patients who developed Hib supraglottitis, 5 of whom had up-to-date Hib vaccination status, suggesting that antibody levels should be measured to identify vaccine failures. Childhood supraglottitis presents as a progressive illness with a toxic-appearing child, classically in a "tripod" position (forward-leaning with extension of the head to maximize airway size).

Adults, on the contrary, have a more gradual course and typically have symptoms of sore throat and odynophagia on presentation. Bizaki and colleagues[13] conducted a retrospective review of 308 cases of adult supraglottitis. The incidence increased more than 2-fold when comparing 1989–1999 to 2000–2009. Sore throat and odynophagia were the most common symptoms. *Streptococcus* was the most common organism identified in throat cultures. Most patients had more than one site involved in the supraglottis, with the epiglottis being most often involved, followed by arytenoids. Fewer than 20% required airway intervention.

When the clinical presentation suggests supraglottitis, priority should be given to securing the airway. In children, attempts at direct visualization or intervention such

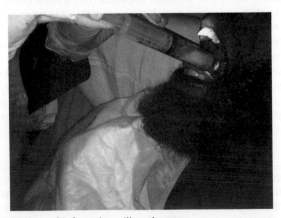

Fig. 11. Needle aspiration of left peritonsillar abscess.

as venipuncture should be delayed until the airway is protected to avoid agitating the patient and causing complete airway obstruction. An "epiglottitis protocol" is activated, whereby the child is rapidly taken to the operating room accompanied by the parent, anesthesiologist, and otolaryngologist. Available equipment should include a tracheotomy set open. Mask induction is undertaken while an intravenous line is inserted. Direct laryngoscopy is performed, which classically demonstrates a "cherry red" epiglottis with edema on the lingual surface resulting in posterior displacement. Once intubation is completed, cultures of the epiglottis are taken, as are blood cultures.

If impending respiratory collapse is not imminent, a lateral neck radiograph may be performed, possibly demonstrating an enlarged epiglottis known as the "thumb sign." Blood cultures should be sent and broad-spectrum antibiotics should be started, most commonly ampicillin-sulbactam or ceftriaxone.[9] More recently, some authors advocate a less aggressive approach to airway intervention and recommend routine use of steroids in addition to intravenous antibiotics.[14]

Adults with supraglottitis rarely have impending airway obstruction; this allows time for evaluation with flexible laryngoscopy to determine the severity of the edema and the need to secure the airway. Serial laryngoscopy may be helpful to ensure that progression has not occurred and could be guided by the patient's symptoms. Video documentation of the laryngoscopic examination may be helpful to allow for a more objective comparison particularly when there has been transfer of care from one physician to another and to permit remote consultation by offsite staff.

If there is significant obstruction initially, or worsening of the obstruction, securing the airway becomes necessary. Awake nasal fiberoptic intubation is indicated when there is adequate visualization of the glottis to allow insertion of the ETT. Preparation must be made for emergent tracheotomy should intubation fail. The Holinger laryngoscope with its prominent curved anterior lip is also an excellent tool for lifting the edematous epiglottis and visualizing the glottis and may be considered an option to secure the airway before emergent tracheotomy. Because of its small lumen, an Eschmann stylet is usually inserted through it first, over which an ETT is passed. This technique does require some experience but will serve as a helpful tool in the armamentarium of airway management (**Fig. 12**). Alternatively, awake tracheotomy could be used as the initial approach.

ANGIOEDEMA

First described in 1882, angioedema, or angioneurotic edema, is characterized by painless, well-circumscribed areas of edema of mucosal or cutaneous surfaces. It is nonpruritic, nonpitting, and nondependent and may involve any part of the body, but has a predilection for the upper aerodigestive tract (**Fig. 13**).[15] It affects up to 10% of the population at some point during their lifetime.[16] A predominance among women and African Americans has been reported in most studies.[17] Angioedema is caused by increased vascular permeability with extravasation of fluid into the submucosal or subcutaneous tissues. The exact mechanisms vary with the different causes, but regardless of the cause, angioedema may quickly progress to life-threatening airway obstruction through oral, pharyngeal, and laryngeal edema and present with challenging airway management scenarios.

Angioedema may be categorized into 2 basic groups: histaminergic or kininergic depending on the pathogenesis.[18] The most common types encountered include anaphylaxis, allergic angioedema without anaphylaxis, angiotensin-converting enzyme (ACE) inhibitor-related angioedema, hereditary angioedema (HAE), and idiopathic angioedema.

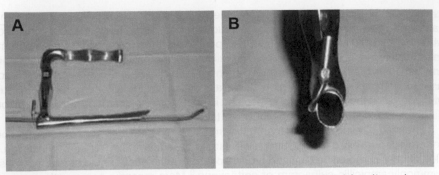

Fig. 12. (A) Holinger laryngoscope lateral view with Eschmann stylet. (B) Holinger laryngo-scope posterior view.

ACE Inhibitor-related Angioedema

ACE inhibitors are widely used medications for the treatment of patients with hyper-tension, congestive heart failure, myocardial infarction, diabetic nephropathy, and chronic kidney disease,[19] and this has resulted in ACE inhibitors being one of the most prescribed medications worldwide.[20] Approximately 35 million to 40 million pre-scriptions were written worldwide in 2001 alone.[21] Consequently, physicians are frequently forced to deal with several adverse effects of this class of medication. Although uncommon, angioedema is a potentially life-threatening adverse effect of ACE inhibitor use. The incidence of ACE inhibitor-related angioedema has been reported to be between 0.1% and 6%.[20,21] Angioedema induced by ACE inhibitors ac-counts for approximately one-third of cases of angioedema encountered in the emer-gency department.[21]

Patients may present with ACE inhibitor-related angioedema anywhere from 1 day to 20 years after starting medication use, and many will have had past self-limited ep-isodes. Presenting symptoms include shortness of breath, dysphagia, odynophagia, stridor, hoarseness, and drooling. Onset of symptoms is usually over several hours and does not include urticaria. The edema is self-limited and typically resolves in 1

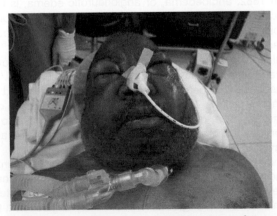

Fig. 13. Patient with angioedema of the face and airway status after tracheotomy.

to 2 days.[20] ACE inhibitor-related angioedema may strike suddenly any time after initiation of ACE inhibitor therapy and no precipitating factors have been identified.[20–23] It is thought that this type of angioedema is primarily caused by the accumulation of bradykinin secondary to inhibition of ACE. As such, ACE inhibitor-related angioedema is a nonhistaminergic angioedema.[20,22] Risk factors found to be associated with ACE inhibitor-related angioedema include the female gender, African American decent, and tobacco use.[21,22] Conversely, diabetes mellitus is associated with a decreased risk of developing this type of angioedema.[24]

Allergic Angioedema

Allergic angioedema is a type of histaminergic angioedema that could be immunoglobulin E–mediated or as a result of direct mast cell degranulation from binding with the allergen. In addition to histamine, there is release or formation of leukotrienes, prostaglandins, tryptase, and other vasoactive peptides; this occurs when there is exposure to a relevant allergen, including foods, stinging insects, latex, and certain drugs. The symptoms are rapid in onset and often include an associated pruritic urticaria, similar to anaphylaxis, which also results from mast cell degranulation, but in which there is also concomitant multisystem involvement, including the lower airways, and the circulatory or gastrointestinal systems. Patients can present at any age and symptoms are rapid in onset, usually less than 1 hour. They are treated with antihistamines and corticosteroids, but if there are any signs of anaphylaxis, epinephrine is also administered. Avoidance of the allergen is advised, and an epinephrine auto injector is prescribed.[25]

Hereditary Angioedema

HAE is a rare autosomal-dominant disorder characterized by repeated episodes of swelling affecting the skin, gastrointestinal tract, face, larynx, and other organs. It is caused in most cases by low levels of functional C1 esterase inhibitor (C1-INH), a serine protease inhibitor that plays important regulatory roles in the complement, contact, and fibrinolytic pathways. Patients often have a positive family history and present with symptoms before the age of 20. There is, in addition however, a rare autosomal-dominant hereditary variety with normal C1-INH levels that is thought to be due to increased bradykinin generation. Acquired C1-INH deficiency has also been reported in patients with underlying lymphoreticular disorders, but will present later in life, usually after 40 years of age.

   Lack of functional C1-INH results in excessive release of bradykinin, which triggers vasodilation, vascular permeability, and edema. Women with HAE present with more frequent and more severe attacks than men as estrogens increase kininogenase activity.[26]

   Most attacks are mild and self-limited, but if left untreated, laryngeal attacks may cause rapid airway obstruction and death. Symptoms are usually gradual over several hours but may also be rapid and progress in less than 1 hour. Potential triggers of laryngeal attacks include trauma to or manipulation of the face, mouth, or upper airway. Therefore, before performing such a procedure in a patient with HAE, there needs to be consultation between the surgeon, the physician managing the HAE, and the anesthesiologist, and appropriate preparations for prevention and/or treatment of an attack need to be made.

   Current World Allergy Organization and European guidelines recommend the use of intravenous plasma-derived C1-INH replacement for short-term prophylaxis of angioedema attacks. Other effective options include danazol given for several days before and after the procedure and fresh-frozen plasma, but these may not be as effective as C1-INH and may be associated with a high rate of adverse events.[27] More recently, icatibant, a bradykinin B2-receptor antagonist, has been shown to be effective in the treatment of acute laryngeal symptoms. A single 30-mg dose of icatibant subcutaneously resulted in symptom improvement in 82% of cases within 1.2 hours with only 5.3% of patients requiring a rescue medication.[28] Patients may also be taught to self-administer the medication at home for recurrent attacks.[29] Ecallantide is a selective reversible inhibitor of plasma kallikrein that reduces the production of bradykinin and has also been shown to be effective in the treatment of laryngeal HAE attacks.[30,31]

Idiopathic Angioedema

The category of idiopathic angioedema includes patients that present with recurrent swelling that may or may not be associated with a pruritic urticaria. Patients may be of any ethnicity and present at any age. It most often affects the lips and tongue but may rarely involve the larynx as well. It may be either mast cell–mediated or bradykinin-related. The former type is more common and responds to antihistamines and corticosteroids. Cases that do not respond to this treatment regimen are quite rare and likely can be categorized into the bradykinin-related category.

Airway Management

Patients with angioedema may present with varying degrees of respiratory distress. Critical to the management of these patients are the history and physical examination, including flexible laryngoscopy. The history will determine the likely cause and guide therapy. Physical examination will reveal a pale "water bag" edema of various sites in the head and neck. In a recent large series of ACE inhibitor-related angioedema, the lips were the most commonly affected site (60.2%), followed by the tongue (39.7%), larynx (29.5%), soft palate/uvula (17%), face (12.5%), and floor of mouth (6.8%). Involvement of multiple sites was present in 48.9% of patients.[32] In a series by Al Khudari and colleagues,[33] angioedema limited to the upper lip was a significant negative predictor of airway edema.

Airway management will range widely depending on the presentation. In mild cases, observation for several hours after medical treatment is adequate. In patients with mild laryngeal edema, serial laryngoscopy is prudent as progression of angioedema was noted by Chan and Soliman[32] in 25% of patients with initially mild laryngeal edema and resulted in intubation. In addition, a stable patient with angioedema who develops new hoarseness or dysphagia should undergo laryngoscopy because these are good positive predictors of laryngeal edema.

In many of these cases, direct laryngoscopy with a Mac or Miller blade and intubation is usually feasible. The GlideScope provides excellent visualization and allows multiple members of the team to view the airway simultaneously; care must be taken to first insert the ETT into the mouth under direct vision until it can be seen on screen to avoid inadvertent injury to the oropharyngeal structures.

Patients with significant floor-of-mouth and/or tongue edema present a challenge because they are not orally intubatable. Significant posterior progression of the edema will result in a situation requiring an emergent surgical airway. Prompt awake fiberoptic nasal intubation is an excellent technique for management of this group as long as the glottis is visible. Awake tracheotomy is recommended if there is involvement of the laryngopharynx compromising access for endotracheal intubation. As always, preintervention discussion and preparation for the initial and contingency airway plans are critical to a successful outcome.

SUMMARY/FUTURE DIRECTIONS

Patients presenting with infections and edema of the head and neck will often have impaired airways. Successful management depends on rapid evaluation, precise diagnosis, and appropriate intervention. A stepwise approach with "Plan A," "Plan B," and "Plan C," and so on is critical in achieving this goal. Simulation laboratories where clinicians can hone their skills and practice working collaboratively have been shown to be effective. Technological advances will reduce their cost and allow for more widespread use.

REFERENCES

1. Bakir S, Tanriverdi MH, Gun R, et al. Deep neck space infections: a retrospective review of 173 cases. Am J Otolaryngol 2012;33(1):56–63.
2. Eftekharian A, Roozbahany NA, Vaezeafshar R, et al. Deep neck infections: a retrospective review of 112 cases. Eur Arch Otorhinolaryngol 2009;266(2):273–7.
3. Staffieri C, Fasanaro E, Favaretto N, et al. Multivariate approach to investigating prognostic factors in deep neck infections. Eur Arch Otorhinolaryngol 2014; 271(7):2061–7.
4. Marra S, Hotaling AJ. Deep neck infections. Am J Otolaryngol 1996;17(5): 287–98.
5. Huang TT, Liu TC, Chen PR, et al. Deep neck infection: analysis of 185 cases. Head Neck 2004;26(10):854–60.
6. Daramola OO, Flanagan CE, Maisel RH, et al. Diagnosis and treatment of deep neck space abscesses. Otolaryngol Head Neck Surg 2009;141(1):123–30.
7. Ridder GJ, Technau-Ihling K, Sander A, et al. Spectrum and management of deep neck space infections: an 8-year experience of 234 cases. Otolaryngol Head Neck Surg 2005;133(5):709–14.
8. Ozbek C, Aygenc E, Tuna E, et al. Use of steroids in the treatment of peritonsillar abscess. J Laryngol Otol 2004;118(6):439–42.
9. Rafei K, Lichenstein R. Airway infectious disease emergencies. Pediatr Clin North Am 2006;53(2):215–42.
10. Stoner MJ, Dulaurier M. Pediatric ENT emergencies. Emerg Med Clin North Am 2013;31(3):795–808.
11. Jenson H. Acute complications of Epstein-Barr virus infectious mononucleosis. Curr Opin Pediatr 2000;12(3):263–8.
12. Shah RK, Roberson DW, Jones DT. Epiglottitis in the hemophilus influenzae type B vaccine era: changing trends. Laryngoscope 2004;114(3):557–60.
13. Bizaki AJ, Numminen J, Laranne J, et al. Acute supraglottitis in adults in Finland: review and analysis of 308 cases. Laryngoscope 2011;121(10):2107–13.
14. Park HH, Lee JC, Kwon JK, et al. Acute supraglottitis in adults: what's the optimal airway intervention? Auris Nasus Larynx 2012;39(2):204–7.
15. Tai S, Mascaro M, Goldstein N. Angioedema: a review of 367 episodes presenting to three tertiary care hospitals. Ann Otol Rhinol Laryngol 2010;119:836–41.
16. Kaplan A. Angioedema. World Allergy Organ J 2008;1(16):103–13.
17. Bentsianov B, Parhiscar A, Azer M, et al. The role of fiberoptic nasopharyngoscopy in the management of the acute airway in angioneurotic edema. Laryngoscope 2000;110(12):2016–9.
18. Moellman JJ, Bernstein JA, Lindsell C, et al. A consensus parameter for the evaluation and management of angioedema in the emergency department. Acad Emerg Med 2014;21(4):469–84.
19. Bickett D. Using ACE inhibitors appropriately. Am Fam Physician 2002;66:461–8.

20. Winters M, Rosenbaum S, Vilke G, et al. Emergency department management of patients with ACE-inhibitor angioedema. J Emerg Med 2013;45:775–80.
21. Banerji A, Clark S, Blanda M, et al. Multicenter study of patients with angiotensin-converting enzyme inhibitor-induced angioedema who present to the emergency department. Ann Allergy Asthma Immunol 2008;100:327–32.
22. Grant N, Deeb Z, Chia S. Clinical experience with angiotensin-converting enzyme inhibitor-induced angioedema. Otolaryngol Head Neck Surg 2007;137:931–5.
23. Piller L, Ford C, Davis B, et al. Incidence and predictors of angioedema in elderly hypertensive patients at high risk for cardiovascular disease: a report from the Antihypertensive and Lipid-Lowering Treatment to Prevent Heart Attack Trial (ALLHAT). J Clin Hypertens 2006;8:649–56.
24. Mahoney E, Devaiah A. Angioedema and angiotensin-converting enzyme inhibitors: are demographics a risk? Otolaryngol Head Neck Surg 2008;139:105–8.
25. Barbara DW, Ronan KP, Maddox DE, et al. Perioperative angioedema: background, diagnosis, and management. J Clin Anesth 2013;25(4):335–43.
26. Bouillet L, Gompel A. Hereditary angioedema in women: specific challenges. Immunol Allergy Clin North Am 2013;33(4):505–11.
27. Bernstein J. Managing hereditary angioedema patients undergoing otolaryngeal procedures. Am J Rhinol Allergy 2013;27(6):522–7.
28. Malbrán A, Riedl M, Ritchie B, et al. Repeat treatment of acute hereditary angioedema attacks with open-label icatibant in the FAST-1 Trial. Clin Exp Immunol 2014;177:544–53.
29. Aberer W. Open-label, multicenter study of self-administered icatibant for attacks of hereditary angioedema. Allergy 2014;69(3):305–14.
30. Sheffer A, MacGinnitie A, Campion M. Outcomes after ecallantide treatment of laryngeal hereditary angioedema attacks. Ann Allergy Asthma Immunol 2013;110:184–8.
31. Berry A, Firszt R. Successful treatment of idiopathic angioedema with ecallantide. J Allergy Clin Immunol Pract 2013;1(3):297–8.
32. Chan N, Soliman A. Angiotensin converting enzyme inhibitor-related angioedema: onset, presentation, and management. Ann Otol Rhinol Laryngol 2015;124:89–96.
33. Al-Khudari S, Loochtan M, Peterson E, et al. Management of angiotensin-converting enzyme inhibitor-induced angioedema. Laryngoscope 2011;121(3):501–2.

Anesthesia Care for the Professional Singer

Ryan K. Meacham, MD*, Joshua Schindler, MD

KEYWORDS

- Anesthesia • Surgery • Voice • Professional singer

KEY POINTS

- Voice is produced by good breath support, smooth vibratory vocal cords for phonation, and an oral cavity for articulation.
- The professional singer should have a detailed informed consent of the risks of anesthesia and/or surgery on the voice.
- Anesthetic considerations include: use smallest possible endotracheal tube or laryngeal mask airway; use low cuff pressure; minimize tube movement; consider corticosteroids and acid reflux prophylaxis.

INTRODUCTION

The administration of anesthesia to a professional voice user warrants special consideration. Whether the patient is a professional singer, actor, radio or TV personality, lawyer, physician, or teacher—all hold exceptional value to their ability to produce voice. To these voice professionals, the ability to produce a clear, strong, and sometimes uniquely distinctive, voice is not only a passion but also a means of livelihood. Therefore this patient may make every effort to protect, conserve, and nurture his or her voice through times of illness, strain, or periods of increased voice demand. To the vocal professional, an upcoming operative procedure requiring anesthesia may be daunting and riddled with anxiety as he or she considers the possible ramifications to the voice.

General anesthesia can affect voice production by interfering with the various components essential for healthy voicing. Voice is produced from a coordinated effort of pulmonary function for adequate breath support, vocal cords capable of phonating with smooth vibratory motion, and an oral cavity that facilitates articulation and resonance. Establishment of an artificial airway and maintenance of general anesthesia may pose risks of altering the voice mechanism postoperatively. This article will focus

Disclosures: The authors have no financial disclosures or conflicts of interest.
Department of Otolaryngology, Oregon Health Sciences University, Portland, OR, USA
* Corresponding author.
E-mail address: ryanmeacham@gmail.com

Anesthesiology Clin 33 (2015) 347–356
http://dx.doi.org/10.1016/j.anclin.2015.02.012
1932-2275/15/$ – see front matter © 2015 Elsevier Inc. All rights reserved.

anesthesiology.theclinics.com

on the application of anesthesia to patients who are professional voice users, with particular attention to the professional singer.

BIOMECHANICS OF VOICE

Although essentially all body systems can directly or indirectly affect the voice, most attention is given to the larynx, the lungs, and the supraglottic vocal tract. For the purposes of this discussion, it is helpful to conceptualize the larynx in 3 main parts: the vocal cords, the intrinsic laryngeal muscles, and the extrinsic laryngeal muscles. From superficial to deep, the vocal cords are composed of an epithelial layer, a superficial lamina propria comprised of gelatinous glycosaminoglycans necessary for smooth vibration of the vocal cords, a vocal ligament extending from the vocal process of the arytenoid cartilage to the anterior commissure, and the muscle bellies of the thyroarytenoid muscle.

As an air column is propelled through the airway, the vocal cords vibrate with smooth and elegant periodicity in an inferior-to-superior manner. Edema or inflammation of the epithelial layer or traumatic injury to the deeper layers of the vocal fold can affect vocal quality. The intrinsic laryngeal muscles adduct and abduct the vocal cords, and the extrinsic laryngeal muscles elevate and depress the larynx (eg, during swallowing). In the trained singer, the extrinsic muscles maintain the larynx in a relatively constant position.[1]

The supraglottic vocal tract is comprised of the supraglottic larynx, the pharynx, the tongue, the hard and soft palates, the nasal cavity, and the sinuses. These structures act in concert to create a resonant chamber, which gives a certain quality to the voice. Alteration of this anatomy with adenotonsillar hypertrophy, growth of nasal polyps, or edema from an upper respiratory infection will invoke changes to the resonance of the voice that may be recognized immediately by the trained vocalist.

In singing, the lungs supply a constant flow of air through the vocal cords and generate the power of a voice. Trained singers generally have an increased efficiency of respiratory use. They do not have an increased total lung capacity as assumed by some, but rather use a higher proportion of air in the lungs, thereby decreasing residual volume.[2]

The abdomen is considered the support system to assist the lungs in maintaining adequate airflow. Although some vocal coaches prefer a distended abdomen, most vocal techniques focus on maintaining the optimal position of the abdomen up and under the rib cage. In each paradigm, an abdominal wall injury is deleterious to the professional voice.

Alterations of the musculoskeletal system may have subtle impacts on the voice. Foot problems may drive the weight of the body to the heels rather than on the metatarsal heads, which in turn increases the strain of abdominal and back musculature enough to affect the voice. Extra tension in the arms and shoulders may cause increased cervical strain and muscle tension dysphonia.

The properly trained singer will assume a favorable position for optimal vocal performance.[1] Surgical intervention on any body part affecting proper vocal technique may have a deleterious impact on the voice mechanism.

PREOPERATIVE CONSIDERATIONS

Treatment of the professional voice user merits careful consideration preoperatively, intraoperatively, and postoperatively (**Table 1**). Appropriate counseling of postoperative expectations should be provided to the professional singer long before the day of surgery. The patient should be provided with realistic expectations about the effects of general anesthesia and intubation on the voice. Following an endotracheal tube intubation, the patient should understand the expected course of mild sore throat, a rough

Table 1	
Anesthetic considerations for the vocal professional	
Preoperative	Detailed informed consent, discussion of risks to the voice
	Consideration of regional anesthesia or LMA
	Gastroesophageal reflux disease (GERD) prophylaxis
	Assessment by otolaryngologist, speech language pathologist
Intraoperative	Direct visualization of intubation, consider videolaryngoscopy
	Use of LMA, or smallest sized endotracheal tube possible
	Most experienced anesthetist to intubate
	Deep muscle relaxation (minimize movement against tube)
	Corticosteroids (decrease vocal cord edema, reduce postoperative nausea and vomiting)
	Close monitoring of cuff pressure, avoid nitrous oxide
	Avoid movement of tube (secure taping, minimize head turns)
	Minimize surgical time
	Deep extubation (avoid bucking on tube)
Postoperative	Set expectations for return of voice
	GERD control
	Possible voice rest
	Assessment by otolaryngologist, speech language pathologist
	Determine timeline of return to performance

or raspy quality to the speaking and singing voice, diminished vocal range, increased voice breaks, globus sensation, and increased throat clearing.

Meticulous documentation of this discussion in the informed consent is prudent for the professional singer. It is important for the record to reflect that the singer has been counseled that voice damage can occur and could leave him or her with a hoarse speaking voice, as well as impaired ability to sing or perform permanently.

According to anesthesia-related claims in a closed claims database, 7% of all claims are related to airway injury.[3] The most frequent site of injury within the airway for anesthesia-related malpractice claims is the larynx, with injuries including vocal cord paralysis, vocal cord hematoma, intubation granulomas, and arytenoid subluxation.[4] These injuries may result in protracted laryngeal dysfunction.[5] Again, these risks should be discussed preoperatively on a visit prior to the day of the operation so that the singer may have time to emotionally prepare and ask relevant questions.

Increased regard to the voice should be provided if the singer is undergoing surgery to the neck, or on the chest or abdomen where postoperative pain may lead to diminished breath support. In these cases, a singer may need to forego performances for several months during full recuperation. For uncomplicated surgery not involving these key body systems, a singer may perform just a few weeks after surgery. Returning to performance prematurely, however, may lead to minor extralaryngeal muscular alterations to compensate for vocal insecurities, and such maladaptive compensations may lead to voice dysfunction in the future.

ANESTHETIC CONSIDERATIONS

Although the consequences of long-term endotracheal tube intubation have been well documented,[6–8] there has been less attention given to the effects of short-term intubation. After short-term intubation, as typically associated with general anesthesia, the experienced listener may detect elements of roughness, strain, breathiness, and weakness to the voice. These effects usually resolve completely within 72 hours; however, the risk of prolonged alteration of the voice is real. Certainly arytenoid dislocation, intubation granuloma, posterior glottic ulceration, and recurrent laryngeal nerve paresis have occurred following intubation and can be devastating to the vocal professional.[9–12] A list of intubation injuries is found in **Table 2**.

Both subjective and objective changes to the voice occur immediately following extubation. Paulauskiene and colleagues[13] evaluated 218 patients preoperatively, 2 hours postoperatively, and 24 hours postoperatively. They found increased symptoms of hoarseness (81%), vocal fatigue (9%), throat clearing (64%), globus pharyngeus (49%), and throat pain (48%) at 2 hours. All of these symptoms improved but were still not at baseline at 24 hours. In their analysis, singing skills of a patient had no impact on the development of these laryngopharyngeal symptoms. Acoustic studies[14–17] have shown that jitter (fluctuation in vocal pitch) and shimmer (fluctuation in vocal intensity) have consistently increased after extubation, while maximum phonation time (ability to sustain a prolonged vowel sound) is decreased, thus underscoring the temporary instability of the voice after extubation.

These acoustic changes may be caused by rheological factors that occur with changes of vocal fold viscosity and stiffness after intubation. Changes to the vibratory characteristics of the vocal folds may occur secondary to alterations in mucosal surface irregularity and abrasions from direct trauma of instrumenting an endotracheal tube. Certainly, vocal fold edema, dehydration, and increased thickened mucus may affect the vibratory capability of the vocal cords and alter the perturbation measures (jitter, shimmer). Anesthetic agents may affect the neuromuscular junction of the laryngeal musculature as well as altering laryngeal sensation, both of which may contribute to altered acoustic measures postoperatively.[18] Decreases in maximum phonation time are secondary to the postanesthetic diminution of breath support, or may be caused by the effects of surgery on the chest or abdomen.

The primary consideration for the anesthesiologist will be the determination of the most appropriate type of airway during the procedure. In select cases, it may be deemed suitable to perform the procedure simply with regional anesthesia. For the vocal professional, he or she may be willing to tolerate more discomfort during surgery if it means foregoing instrumentation of the larynx. Certainly, this should be a collaborative decision between the patient, surgeon, and anesthesia provider.

In cases in which establishment of an airway is necessary, endotracheal tube or laryngeal mask airway may be the primary means of ventilation. Each of these types of artificial airway has its own advantages and risks to the voice.

Endotracheal Tube

There has been some discussion on the preferable route of intubation to minimize trauma to the larynx. Opinion has varied whether a nasotracheal route decreases tube motion and allows less mucosal ulceration in the larynx, or if greater endotracheal

Table 2 Intubation injuries affecting the voice	
Vocal Fold Injuries	Abrasion
	Laceration
	Hematoma
	Granuloma
	Paralysis
Cartilage Injuries	Cricoarytenoid dislocation
Stenotic Injuries	Posterior glottic stenosis
	Subglottic stenosis

tube flexibility during orotracheal intubation is less likely to cause injury. Data regarding the superiority of the nasotracheal route have been mixed.

In a small study of 17 patients intubated in the intensive care unit (ICU) for an average of 7 days, Dubick and Wright[19] performed laryngoscopy at the time of extubation or tracheostomy tube placement and found a higher incidence of injury to the vocal cords and laryngeal cartilages in those patients who had been intubated via an orotracheal route versus a nasotracheal route, presumably due to less movement of the nasotracheal tube. However, Colice and colleagues[20] examined 82 patients who were equally divided among orotracheal and nasotracheal intubations and found no difference in laryngeal injury.

A good rule of thumb in the professional singer for the anesthesia provider is to not deviate far from the usual (and safe) way of practicing anesthesia. Thus, if one has less experience performing nasotracheal intubation, it would not be prudent to attempt it for the professional singer.

In a survey of members of the Voice Foundation (primarily otolaryngologists with an emphasis in treating voice disorders), several recommendations were noted in regard to the intubation of professional singers.[21] A majority (76%) favored a smaller endotracheal tube for singers (6.0 for females, 6.0 or 7.0 for males) via the oral (46%) versus the nasal (36%) route. Personally, the authors of this article favor a 5.0 or 5.5 tube when possible.

Emergence from anesthesia may be just as key as induction in preventing laryngeal trauma. A deep extubation followed by masking may prevent the patient from coughing and bucking against the tube. If the tube is left in place during emergence, it is helpful to untape the tube to allow it to move up and down when the patient swallows rather than be a fixed tube that rubs and possibly abrades the vocal folds with laryngeal movement.

Laryngeal Mask Airway

The laryngeal mask airway (LMA) was introduced in the United Kingdom by Dr Brain in 1983.[22] In routine use, a laryngoscope is not required for placement of the LMA, and its uses have been shown to be applicable to many aspects of anesthesia care, except where regurgitation of gastric contents is probable. LMA may be considered in the professional singer in order to avoid instrumentation of the vocal cords or subglottis.

Removal of the LMA with an inflated cough, forced traction, or twisting of the LMA may cause rotation of the larynx and possible arytenoid dislocation. Several cranial nerve injuries arising from pressure-induced neuropraxia have been attributed to use of the LMA. One review found reports of LMA-associated neuropathies of the lingual nerve (6 cases), hypoglossal nerve (6 cases), and recurrent laryngeal nerve (11 cases).[23] Diffusion of nitrous oxide into the LMA cuff causing increased cuff pressures has been implicated as a culprit.[24]

Although the LMA does not directly traumatize the vocal cords, it cannot completely absolve itself of any laryngeal damage whatsoever. High cuff pressures may seal the mask against the supraglottis, causing postoperative edema and alteration of the supraglottic vocal tract. Furthermore, dessication of the vocal folds may occur secondary to the constant blow-by of anesthetic gases. This may lead to an increase in the adhesiveness of the vocal folds during phonation and subsequent dysphonia.[25]

Medications

Muscle relaxation with paralytic agents should be used routinely in the anesthesia management of the professional singer. Increased paralysis leads to less motion of the tube against the larynx. Motion created by neck flexion/extension, coughing, gagging, swallowing, and tongue movement may abrade the laryngeal mucosa and lead to ulcerations. In 1 study, those patients that were maintained in a flaccid state had less laryngeal injury,[20] while it was found in a separate report that head trauma patients with rigid posturing had an increased incidence of laryngeal damage.[26]

Although glycopyrrolate may be helpful to decrease oral and respiratory secretions to aid in an unobstructed view for an atraumatic intubation, the anticholinergic properties may lead to undesirable consequences on the voice. The drying effect may result in decreased vocal cord lubrication, increased throat clearing, and frequent coughing.

Corticosteroids should probably be administered intraoperatively to all nondiabetic professional vocalists, because they decrease edema of the vocal cords. The evidence behind this recommendation, however, is lacking.

Other Factors

It is intuitive that the duration of anesthesia and the number of intubation attempts may result in increased voice complaints following surgery, which has been demonstrated in some[27,28] but not all[29] reports. One randomized controlled trial compared the inflation of an endotracheal tube cuff with air or saline and analyzed the incidence of hoarseness and sore throat in ICU patients.[30] Although they found that cuffs inflated with air increased more (presumably to inward diffusion of nitrous oxide) than cuffs with saline, there was no difference in the incidence of hoarseness or sore throat.

The Paulauskiene report[13] demonstrated that tube cuff pressure and volume were related to postoperative voice complaints at 2 and 24 hours after extubation, and this finding was confirmed by Hamdan.[31] When the volume of the cuff increases, the contact area of the cuff and trachea increases, and if cuff pressures exceed the capillary perfusion pressure of 39 cm H_2O, mucosal necrosis occurs followed by tissue sloughing and subglottic stenosis. Cuff pressures should ideally be maintained at 20 to 25 cm H_2O, or the lowest pressure that allows adequate ventilation.

SURGICAL CONSIDERATIONS

Otolaryngologists are frequently queried about the effects of tonsillectomy on the voice. After removal of the palatine tonsils, the supraglottic vocal tract is anatomically reconfigured, and the size of the resonant chamber increases, thus altering voice.[32,33] Furthermore, scarring of the tonsillar beds can reduce pharyngeal contracture; although this may be an imperceptible change to the casual voice user, it can noticeably affect the professional singer. Notwithstanding these changes, 1 study of healthy (nonsinger) children found that some acoustic measurements may actually improve after tonsillectomy.[34] Singers must undoubtedly be cautioned that their voice may change following tonsillectomy. It may take 3 to 6 months following tonsillectomy for a singer's voice to approach its new baseline.[1]

Surgery anywhere along the course of the fibers of the recurrent laryngeal nerve may lead to vocal cord paralysis. Surgery of the brainstem, skull base, neck, and chest all may lead to an untoward neurologic paralysis and dysphonia. Thyroid surgery places both the recurrent laryngeal nerve and the external branch of the superior laryngeal nerve at risk. Injury to the superior laryngeal nerve will result in decreased vocal range, as the cricothyroid muscle is unable to elongate and tense the vocal fold. Division of the strap muscles during thyroidectomy may lead to increased extralaryngeal scarring and destabilization of the laryngeal skeleton.

Thoracic and abdominal surgery may interfere with respiratory support. Singers should be cautioned against singing until surgical pain has subsided. Premature introduction to performance without proper breath support will invariably lead to increased cervical muscle tension as the singer attempts to power through the voice via an unsupported system. One author requires that the singer be able to do 10 sit-ups prior to resuming singing after thoracic or abdominal surgery.[35] Other surgeries may negatively impact vocal function if they alter the stance of the singer or otherwise affect the musculoskeletal system.

POSTOPERATIVE CONSIDERATIONS

Close follow-up after surgery is judicious for the professional singer. Hoarseness may be noted after surgery, and a plan for further care can be established. Certainly, if the patient is admitted following surgery, it is wise for the anesthesia provider to make a postoperative visit and document the current state of the voice. It is imperative that the vocalist not feel abandoned during this time when he or she feels vulnerable.

Consultation with an otolaryngologist, particularly a laryngology voice specialist, may be advisable following general anesthesia and surgery when hoarseness persists more than a few days after surgery. Visualization of the vocal folds via fiber optic laryngoscopy is particularly useful to evaluate the condition of the larynx, and vocal folds in particular. Vocal cord hematomas from traumatic intubation may necessitate voice rest. Small abrasions of the mucosal covering of the vocal fold may be best treated with added humidification. Vocal fold paresis or paralysis from a temporary intubation neuropraxia or surgical injury may be observed for improvement or may merit an injection laryngoplasty with a temporary injectable filler while waiting for return of nerve function. The rare case of cricoarytenoid joint subluxation may warrant an examination under anesthesia.

For most cases of postsurgical dysphonia, the evaluation and treatment by a speech language pathologist proves invaluable. Reintroduction of proper vocal technique to the professional singer is key to avoid maladaptive behaviors that may result in muscle tension dysphonia to compensate for an altered voice mechanism. A trusted voice teacher with close knowledge of the singer's instrument is invaluable during this period.

Transient postextubation aspiration is considered common, although usually for just a short duration.[36,37] Acid reflux with resultant laryngeal edema may contribute to laryngeal dysfunction and aspiration.[20] For the professional singer, 1 week of postoperative proton pump inhibitor therapy may provide a notable benefit. Mucolytic agents assist in thinning mucus secretions and may alleviate cough and throat clearing. Postoperative corticosteroids should not be given as a matter of routine, but should be considered to facilitate recovery of prolonged vocal fold edema or acute laryngitis, particularly in the performer with an imminent performance. Aspirin and other anticoagulants should be avoided if possible in the perioperative period, as they can predispose to vocal cord hemorrhage.

In the case of the professional singer, there may be pressure to recover expeditiously from surgery if a performance date looms near. Certainly it is ideal if the performer has no commitments for performance dates at the time of surgery; this way, the vocalist will not rush back and risk damage to the voice. If the surgery is relatively minor, and the intubation was not traumatic to the larynx, the singer could return to performing as soon as 1 week following surgery (**Fig. 1**). However, if surgery involves the neck, chest, or abdomen, or if there is any concern about the condition of the larynx, coordination with an otolaryngologist is recommended for further planning, and a performing hiatus of several months may be necessary.

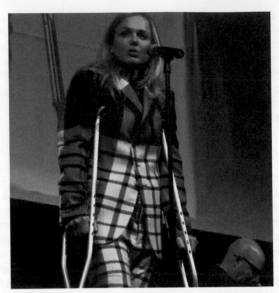

Fig. 1. Storm Large performs 3 days after general anesthesia for surgery on a lower extremity. (*Courtesy of* Storm Large, Portland, OR.)

SUMMARY

The professional singer holds particular value to his or her voice. The professional singer will make every effort to preserve the quality and nature of his or her voice. The anesthesiologist must be prepared to counsel these patients preoperatively about the risks of anesthesia to the voice, and then be prepared to finely tune the delivery of anesthesia to both optimize the safety of the procedure as well as minimize the risks of anesthesia to the voice. An understanding of these principles will ensure the protection of the voice postoperatively and expedite the speedy return to normal vocal function.

REFERENCES

1. Sataloff RT. Professional singers: the science and art of clinical care. Am J Otolaryngol 1981;2(3):251–66.
2. Gould WJ, Okamura H. Static lung volumes in singers. Ann Otol Rhinol Laryngol 1973;82:89–95.
3. Metzner J, Posner KL, Lam MS, et al. Closed claims' analysis. Best Pract Res Clin Anaesthesiol 2011;25(2):263–76.
4. Domino KB, Posner KL, Caplan RA, et al. Airway injury during anesthesia: a closed claims analysis. Anesthesiology 1999;91(6):1703–11.
5. Colice GL. Resolution of laryngeal injury following translaryngeal intubation. Am Rev Respir Dis 1992;145(2, pt 1):361–4.
6. McGovern FH, Fitz-Hugh GS, Edgemon LJ. The hazards of endotracheal intubation. Ann Otol Rhinol Laryngol 1981;80:556.
7. Hedden M, Ersoz CJ, Donnelly HW, et al. Laryngotracheal damage after prolonged use of orotracheal tubes in adults. JAMA 1977;207:703.
8. Weymuller E, Bishop M. Problems associated with prolonged intubation in the geriatric patient. Otolaryngol Clin North Am 1990;23:1057–74.

9. Peppard S, Dickens J. Laryngeal injury following short term intubation. Ann Otol Rhinol Laryngol 1983;92:327–30.
10. Keane W, Rowe L, Denneny J, et al. Complications of intubation. Ann Otol Rhinol Laryngol 1982;91:584–7.
11. Balestrieri F, Watson C. Intubation granuloma. Otolaryngol Clin North Am 1982; 15:567–79.
12. Gallivan G, Dawson J, Opfell A. Videolaryngoscopy after endotracheal intubation. Part II: a critical care perspective of lesions affecting voice. J Voice 1990;4: 159–64.
13. Paulauskiene I, Lesinkas E. Laryngopharyngeal complaints following short-term endotracheal intubation: peculiarities of males and females. Acta Medica Lituanica 2012;19(2):51–7.
14. Horii Y, Fuller B. Selected acoustic characteristics of voices before intubation and after extubation. J Speech Lang Hear Res 1990;33:505–10.
15. Beckford NS, Mayo R, Wilkinson A III, et al. Effects of short endotracheal intubation on vocal function. Laryngoscope 1990;100:331–6.
16. Lesser TH, Williams RG, Hoddinott C. Laryngographic changes following endotracheal intubation in adults. Br J Disord Commun 1986;21:239–44.
17. Gleeson MJ, Fourcin AJ. Clinical analysis of laryngeal trauma secondary to intubation. J R Soc Med 1983;76:928.
18. Cohen RL, MacKenzie AI. Anesthesia and cognitive functioning. Anaesthesia 1982;37:47–52.
19. Dubick MN, Wright BD. Comparison of laryngeal pathology following long-term oral and nasal endotracheal intubations. Anesth Analg 1978;57:663–8.
20. Colice GL, Stukel TA, Dain B. Laryngeal complications of prolonged intubation. Chest 1989;96:877–84.
21. Powner DJ. Airway considrations for professional singers—a survey of expert opinion. J Voice 2002;16(4):488–94.
22. Brain AI. The laryngeal mask—a new concept in airway management. Br J Anaesth 1983;55:801–5.
23. Brimacombe J, Clarke G, Keller C. Lingual nerve injury associated with the ProSeal laryngeal mask airway: a case report and review of the literature. Br J Anaesth 2005;95(3):420–3.
24. Bruce IA, Ellis R, Kay NJ. Nerve injury and the laryngeal mask airway. J Laryngol Otol 2004;118(11):899–901.
25. Jiang J, Verdolini K, Aquino B, et al. Effects of dehydration on phonation in excised canine larynges. Ann Otol Rhinol Laryngol 2000;109:568–75.
26. Dunham CM, LaMonica C. Prolonged tracheal intubation in the trauma patient. J Trauma 1984;24:120–4.
27. Kloub R. Sore throat following tracheal intubation. Middle East J Anesthesiol 2001;1:29–40.
28. Rieger A, Brunne B, Hass I, et al. Laryngo-pharyngeal complaints following laryngeal mask airway and endotracheal intubation. J Clin Anesth 1997;9: 42–7.
29. Christensen AM, Willemoes-Larsen H, Lundby L, et al. Postoperative throat complaints after tracheal intubation. Br J Anaesth 1994;73:786–7.
30. Bennett MH, Isert PR, Cumming RG. Postoperative sore throat and hoarseness following tracheal intubation using air or saline to inflate the cuff—a randomized controlled trial. Anaesth Intensive Care 2000;28:408–13.
31. Hamdan AL, Sibai A, Rameh C, et al. Short-term effects of endotracheal intubation on voice. J Voice 2007;21(6):762–8.

32. Gould WJ, Alberti PW, Brodnitz F, et al. Medical care preventive therapy (panel). In: Lawrence V, editor. Transcripts of the seventh annual symposium, care of the professional voice, vol. 3. New York: The Voice Foundation; 1978. p. 74–6.
33. Wallner LJ, Hill BJ, Waldrop W, et al. Voice changes following adenotonsillectomy. Laryngoscope 1968;78:1410–8.
34. Salami A, Jankowska B, Dellepiane M, et al. The impact of tonsillectomy with or without adenoidectomy on speech and voice. Int J Pediatr Otorhinolaryngol 2008; 72(9):1377–84.
35. Sataloff RT. The professional voice. Otolaryngol Head Neck Surg 1991;3: 2029–56.
36. Conlan AA, Kopec SE. Tracheostomy in the ICU. J Intensive Care Med 2000;15: 1–13.
37. Loucks TM, Duff D, Wong JH, et al. The vocal athlete and endotracheal intubation: a management protocol. J Voice 1998;12:349–59.

The Role of Cricothyrotomy, Tracheostomy, and Percutaneous Tracheostomy in Airway Management

CrossMark

Jason A. Akulian, MD, MPH[a], Lonny Yarmus, DO[b],
David Feller-Kopman, MD[c],*

KEYWORDS

- Cricothyrotomy • Airway management • Percutaneous dilational tracheostomy
- Surgical tracheostomy

KEY POINTS

- Cricothyrotomy (CRIC), percutaneous dilational tracheostomy (PDT), and surgical tracheostomy (ST) placement are important means of securing an artificial airway in patients with acute or chronic respiratory failure.
- Use of CRIC or ST is effective in acute/emergency upper airway obstruction, allowing establishment of an airway in cannot intubate/cannot oxygenate scenarios.
- PDT and ST are safe and cost-effective procedures performed on patients requiring prolonged mechanical ventilation, typically in the intensive care setting.
- A growing body of literature has demonstrated that PDT is not only equivalent in outcomes, but may in fact be a superior modality.

INTRODUCTION

The establishment of an artificial airway by means of surgical incision is a procedure dating to the 36th century BC Egypt.[1] A more famous example from antiquity is its

Conflicts of Interest: There were no contract, funding or conflicts of interest involved in the writing of this article.
[a] Section of Interventional Pulmonology, Division of Pulmonary and Critical Care Medicine, University of North Carolina at Chapel Hill, 8007 Burnett Womack, CB 7219, Chapel Hill, NC 27599-7219, USA; [b] Section of Interventional Pulmonology, Division of Pulmonary and Critical Care, Johns Hopkins Hospital, Johns Hopkins University, 1800 Orleans Street, Suite 7125, Baltimore, MD 21287, USA; [c] Bronchoscopy and Interventional Pulmonology, Section of Interventional Pulmonology, Division of Pulmonary and Critical Care Medicine, Johns Hopkins Hospital, Johns Hopkins University, Baltimore, MD 21287, USA
* Corresponding author.
E-mail address: dfellerk@jhmi.edu

Anesthesiology Clin 33 (2015) 357–367
http://dx.doi.org/10.1016/j.anclin.2015.02.009
anesthesiology.theclinics.com

performance by Alexander the Great (356–323 BC), who was reported to have performed a tracheostomy on a choking soldier in his army, "…opened the trachea of a choking soldier with the point of his sword."

Over the ensuing 2500 years, the practice was variously reported and refined, yet seemed to fall out of favor until the 16th century, when Italian surgeon Antonia Brasavola performed the procedure on a patient dying from asphyxiation from an upper airway obstruction and is quoted as saying, "…when there is no other possibility, in angina, of admitting air to the heart, we must incise the larynx below the abscess."[2]

It was not until the early 20th century that placement of artificial airways regained popularity after standardization of the open surgical technique by Chevalier Jackson. Jackson's standardization of the surgical tracheostomy (ST) technique is credited with reducing the operative mortality associated with tracheotomy at that time from 25% to 1%. He recognized and emphasized the importance of adequate oxygenation during the procedure, as well as maintaining control of the airway. He also further advanced all surgical techniques by recognizing the importance of postoperative care. In the 1930s, tracheostomy was advocated as an effective way to provide adequate bronchopulmonary toilet in patients with polio. Because of the continued modern track record of safety associated with ST along with the widespread use of positive pressure ventilation in the 1950s, there was considerable effort focused on the development of tracheostomy tubes as a means of providing long-term ventilatory support.[2] Following this era, cricothyrotomy (CRIC) and percutaneous dilational tracheostomy (PDT) were introduced as alternative techniques. Although these techniques have not replaced ST, they have been shown to be safe and effective. This has led to a growing body of literature attempting to parse out which patients would benefit most from each individual technique. This article discusses each technique, its indications, contraindications, complications, and the comparative data.

CRICOTHYROTOMY
History of Cricothryrotomy

First described in 1805, then successfully performed in 1852, CRIC was introduced long after the first tracheostomy was performed. Initially championed by Chevelier Jackson, who in 1909 described the surgical technique and considerations to successfully perform the procedure, he later abandoned the technique after publishing a case series of 200 patients with post-CRIC tracheal stenosis.[3] In 1976, Brantigan published a case series of 655 patients in which the overall complication rate was 6.1%, with only 8 patients developing tracheal stenosis, 5 of whom required resection of the lesions.[4] This publication combined with subsequent case series reporting low rates of postsurgical complication again popularized the procedure as a method of emergency airway management.

CURRENT TECHNIQUES FOR CRICOTHYROTOMY
Surgical Cricothyrotomy

Surgical CRIC (SCRIC) is performed by identifying the cricothyroid membrane and immobilizing the larynx. Once done, a vertical incision is made first cutaneously, then horizontally through the cricothyroid membrane. A tracheal hook is then inserted superiorly and is used to lift the thyroid cartilage. The incision is dilated using forceps, and a small endotracheal or tracheostomy tube is inserted into the distal airway and fixed in place. A modified 4-step technique involves incision of both the skin and cricothryoid membrane in a single horizontal motion followed by insertion of the tracheal hook inferiorly stabilizing the trachea. The endotracheal or tracheostomy tube is then placed and secured.

Although randomized data concerning technique superiority are lacking, animal and cadaveric studies have shown the 4-step technique to be faster but associated with increased complications.[5–7]

Percutaneous Cricothyrotomy

Percutaneous CRIC (PCRIC) employs the modified Seldinger technique to cannulate the trachea. After a small skin incision is made, an introducer needle is inserted into the airway with verification of entry into the trachea by free aspiration of air; a wire is then inserted via the needle. The needle is then removed, and the insertion site is enlarged via a scalpel incision. The PCRIC tube with dilator is then inserted over the wire with subsequent removal of the dilator and wire en bloc. Upon removal of the dilator and wire, the tube is fixed in place.

Like the different SCRIC methods, randomized controlled trials comparing SCRIC with PCRIC are lacking, as these procedures are typically performed in emergent settings. Cadaveric studies have shown conflicting results in regards to procedural speed, success, and complication rates.[6,8–10]

Needle Cricothyrotomy

Needle CRIC (NCRIC) utilizes a cannula over a needle attached to a suction syringe. The needle is used to puncture the skin, connective tissue, and cricothyroid membrane. Once air is aspirated, indicating entry into the trachea, the cannula is passed forward and into the trachea; the needle is then removed, and the cannula is fixed in place.

INDICATIONS, CONTRAINDICATIONS, AND COMPLICATIONS OF CRICOTHYROTOMY

The primary indication for CRIC is an inability to maintain airway patency/control using standard airway techniques (bag mask, laryngeal mask airway, or endotracheal intubation) during episodes of respiratory failure, particularly in the setting of upper airway compromise.[11–14] The most important contraindication to CRIC placement is the lack of need or the ability to maintain the airway using standard techniques. Other contraindications, both relative and absolute, primarily involve damage or distortion of the site of insertion. Both acute and chronic CRIC complications have been recognized and include loss of the airway, bleeding, posterior tracheal injury, and subglottic stenosis.[15–20] **Table 1** details a complete accounting of contraindications and

Table 1	
Cricothyrotomy contraindications and complications	
Relative Contraindications	**Complications**
Tracheal transection	Bleeding

Laryngotracheal disruption
Retraction of the distal trachea into the mediastinum
Fractured larynx
Pediatric patients
	Laceration of:
	  Thyroid cartilage
	  Cricoid cartilage
	  Tracheal rings

Bleeding diathesis	Posterior tracheal injury
Operator inexperience	False tract
Insertion site infection	Infection
	Tracheostomy tube cuff rupture
Absolute Contraindications	Decannulation
None	Subglottic stenosis
	Voice changes

complications associated with CRIC placement. It should be noted that in the case of complete upper airway obstruction, it may be difficult/impossible to ventilate patients via small-bore CRIC tubes, and in these cases, the tubes are initially inserted to provide oxygenation while a more definitive airway is obtained.

HISTORY OF PERCUTANEOUS DILATIONAL TRACHEOSTOMY

Performance of PDT was first reported in 1955 by Shelden and colleagues,[21] whose initial report described a technique that could provide a rapidly obtained and stable airway in patients with severe head trauma. Their method involved a fixation needle, finder needle and cutting trocar, which introduced the tracheostomy tube. Reports of injuries to the trachea and aorta related to the new technique suggested that the force required to place the tracheostomy via this method may have led to adverse outcomes.[22,23] Toye and Weinstein[24] presented a similar device in 1969 that combined dilation and cutting into 1 instrument with the addition of a guide wire; however, the technique was never widely adopted. The modern PDT era began when Ciaglia published his experience using serial tracheal dilations over a wire in 1985.[25]

CURRENT TECHNIQUES FOR PERCUTANEOUS DILATIONAL TRACHEOSTOMY

No consensus for performing PDT exists. However, standard practice is to perform the procedure on electively paralyzed patients under general anesthesia with bronchoscopic guidance. This is done to reduce the risk of posterior tracheal injury.[26] When possible, the patient is positioned with the neck hyperextended, and the pretrachea is evaluated for vessels traversing the working space. The cricoid and laryngeal cartilages are palpated, and an insertion site between the second and third tracheal ring is selected. After creation of a sterile field, the skin and subcutaneous tissue are infiltrated with lidocaine with epinephrine to promote hemostasis and provide some immediate postprocedure analgesia. Insertion is then performed using one of the following techniques.

The Cialgia Technique

Ciaglia and colleagues[25] first reported their percutaneous technique in 1985 using a modified percutaneous nephrostomy tube placement setup. The originally proposed insertion site for the tracheostomy tube was the space separating the cricoid cartilage and first tracheal ring or the first intertracheal ring space. The site was identified by palpation and an incision made. After blunt dissection, the endotracheal tube (ETT) was withdrawn to a point immediately distal to the vocal cords. A needle was then used to puncture the trachea, and the ETT was manipulated. If the needle moved with ETT movement, the process was repeated after further retraction of the ETT tube until there was no movement of the needle with ETT manipulation, and air flowed freely through the needle. A cannula was then inserted followed by a guide wire and dilation with several additional dilators. Finally, the tracheostomy tube was introduced over a dilator and secured in place.

The original technique has been further refined since its first report with regard to the dilation method and site placement. Commercially available kits include the Smiths-Portex PDT UniPerc (Smiths Medical, Dublin, Ohio), or the Ciaglia Blue Rhino single dilation (BRPDT) (Cook Medical, Bloomington, Indiana) and Ciaglia Blue Dolphin (Cook Medical) (Fig. 1). These kits have replaced serial dilation with a single hydrophilic dilator or an expandable balloon for dilation, respectively. Two small single-center, randomized trials comparing the BRPDT kit with traditional multiple dilation kits found that the single dilation technique with the BRPDT resulted in shorter procedure times and

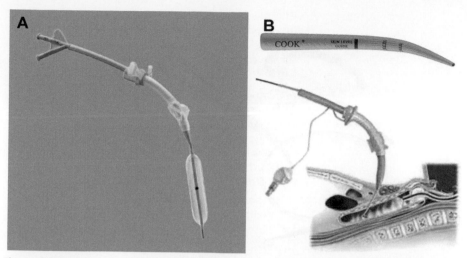

Fig. 1. (*A*) Blue Dolphin percutaneous dilational tracheostomy introducer. (*B*) Blue Rhino percutaneous dilational tracheostomy introducer and procedure illustration. (*Courtesy of Cook Medical Inc, Bloomington, IN; with permission.*)

was not associated with an increase in the complication rate.[27,28] A large multicenter study of 500 consecutive patients with a before-and-after design found a decrease in complication rates after switching the multiple dilator to a single-insertion technique (13.6%–6.5%).[29]

In a recent, small, single-center, randomized comparison of the BRPDT and Blue Dolphin, Cianchi and colleagues,[30] found a longer procedure time, increased incidence of difficulty passing the tracheostomy tube, and an increased risk of minor bleeding associated with use of the Blue Dolphin kit.

The Griggs Technique

In 1994, Griggs and colleagues,[31] introduced a new PDT technique, which substituted a modified Howard-Kelly forceps—the Griggs forceps—designed to slide over a guide wire for the serial dilators used in the Ciaglia method (**Fig. 2**). The initial portion of the procedure is identical to the Ciaglia method in terms of patient preparation, position, initial incision, finder cannula placement, and guide wire placement. After removing the Seldinger needle and after passage of the guide wire into the trachea, the Griggs forceps are passed over the wire and used to dilate the pretracheal soft tissues and then the tracheal tissues to the appropriate diameter. A tracheostomy tube is then inserted over the wire loaded on an appropriately sized dilator. Two single-center prospective trials comparing the original serial Ciaglia dilation technique with the Griggs technique both found that the serial dilation technique took longer than the Griggs' technique.[32,33] The small, nonrandomized trial did not find any statistically significant differences in complication rates between the 2 methods.[32] The larger, randomized trial found an increase in minor and major complications (including pneumothorax, posterior tracheal injury, loss of a stable airway, and conversion to a different procedure) using the progressive dilation method.[33] Several randomized, longitudinal trials comparing the single dilation Ciaglia technique and the Griggs technique have also been conducted.[34–38] A meta-analysis of these trials found evidence of superiority of the Ciaglia technique using a combined endpoint representing procedural difficulties and bleeding.[39]

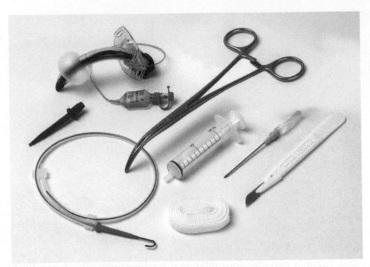

Fig. 2. UniPerc adjustable flange extended-length tracheostomy tubes. (*Courtesy of* Smiths Medical, Dublin, OH; with permission.)

INDICATIONS, CONTRAINDICATIONS AND COMPLICATIONS OF PERCUTANEOUS DILATIONAL TRACHEOSTOMY

Percutaneous tracheostomy is typically reserved for patients who are unable to wean from mechanical ventilation. PDT is generally not considered as the initial airway of choice when faced with a "cannot intubate cannot ventilate" situation. The timing of PDT remains controversial with conflicting data regarding early versus late tracheostomy.[40–47] It should be noted, however, that at least 1 publication has put PDT forward as an emergency airway option.[48] Relative contraindications for PDT include but are not limited to uncorrectable coagulopathy, inability to extend the neck, c-spine instability, aberrant neck vasculature, distortion of the anterior tracheal anatomy, and overlying cellulitis. Although safe and effective, PDT is not without risk. Of complications known to be associated with PDT, trachea-innominate artery fistulas and posterior tracheal injury tend to be the most feared.[49–51] Other rare complications include loss of the airway during placement, errant placement of the tracheostomy tube, subcutaneous emphysema, pneumomediastinum, pneumothorax, infection, tracheal stenosis, significant bleeding, and death.[52–54] As with other procedures, prevention is paramount, and the risks of performing PDT on the critically ill patient should be weighed carefully against the benefits. The proceduralist should carefully consider the ventilator settings, coagulation parameters, airway land marks, hemodynamics, and integrity of the superficial tissue prior to proceeding with PDT. **Table 2** details the contraindications and complications associated with tracheostomy placement.

HISTORY AND INDICATION FOR SURGICAL TRACHEOSTOMY

Performance of open ST is a time-honored procedure[55] involving incision and dissection of the soft tissue overlying the anterior trachea followed by either removal of the anterior segment of a tracheal ring or creation of a tracheal flap, after which a tracheostomy tube is placed into the trachea and fixed in place. Historically used in the treatment of upper airway obstruction, ST has become predominantly used in the treatment of

Table 2
Tracheostomy contraindications and complications

Relative Contraindications	Complications
Uncorrectable coagulopathy/thrombocytopenia	Bleeding
Difficult airway	Pneumothorax
Morbid obesity (PDT only)	Pneumomediastinum
High positive end expiratory pressure	Esophageal injury
Pediatric population	Laryngeal nerve injury
Recent sternotomy	Posterior tracheal injury
History of neck surgery (PDT only)	False tract
Emergent airway (PDT only)	Infection
	Tracheostomy tube cuff rupture
Absolute Contraindications	Decannulation
Insertion site infection	Subglottic stenosis
Operator inexperience	Voice changes
Infants (PDT only)	Tracheo-innominate artery fistula
	Tracheo-esophageal fistula
	Tracheal stenosis
	Granulation tissue

those patients unable to wean from mechanical ventilation who are deemed to be poor candidates for PDT, or following resection of head and neck cancer.

CONTRAINDICATIONS AND COMPLICATIONS IN SURGICAL TRACHEOSTOMY

The contraindications in ST are essentially the same as those for PDT, except for patients having undergone recent sternotomy. Common thought among physicians is that patients who have either poor neck architecture, aberrant vasculature or difficult to correct coagulopathies, or who are dependent on positive end expiratory pressure (PEEP) are more appropriate for ST. Complications for ST are also the same as those for PDT (see **Table 2**).

Surgical Tracheostomy Versus Cricothyrotomy

Few data exist comparing these techniques, again likely because of the emergent nature of CRIC placement. In 2 retrospective case series, severity and timing of complications were found to be similar when comparing the techniques, with the tracheostomy far more commonly performed.[56,57]

Surgical Tracheostomy Versus Percutaneous Dilational Tracheostomy

Since its introduction, many studies including meta-analyses have been published demonstrating the equivalence and even potential superiority of PDT over ST in suitable patients.[58–61] The 2 most recent and statistically robust meta-analyses included over 1000 patients, with both showing a significant reduction in the risk of wound infection and length of procedure time associated with PDT. In addition, no difference in bleeding risk or mortality was noted when comparing modalities.[59,60] One of the 2 meta-analyses found an increased risk of decannulation and obstruction associated with PDT. The authors noted, however, that complication severity was not recorded or reported.[60]

Cost has been shown to be one of the most strongly differentiating factors between PDT and surgical tracheostomy. In a single-center prospective evaluation of cost-effectiveness using charge generation as a surrogate for cost, Freeman and colleagues,[62] showed significantly decreased costs associated with PDT. In a large meta-analysis, Higgins and Punthakee,[60] also found decreased cost associated with PDT. Several authors have suggested that a substantial portion of the cost savings associated with PDT results from avoidance of the operating room and its associated costs.[62,63]

SUMMARY

CRIC, PDT, and ST placement are all important means of securing an artificial airway in patients with acute or chronic respiratory failure. Use of CRIC or ST is effective in acute/emergency upper airway obstruction, allowing establishment of an airway in cannot intubate cannot oxygenate scenarios. PDT and ST are safe and cost-effective procedures performed on patients requiring prolonged mechanical ventilation, typically in the intensive care setting. Although ST has been performed over a much longer period of time, a growing body of literature has demonstrated that PDT is not only equivalent in outcomes, but may in fact be a superior modality, both in regards to outcomes and cost-effectiveness when applied in the correct patient population.

REFERENCES

1. Durbin CG Jr. Techniques for performing tracheostomy. Respir Care 2005;50(4): 488–96.
2. Yarmus LB. Principles and practice of interventional pulmonology. 1st edition. New York: Springer; 2012.
3. Mace SE, Hedges JR. Cricothyrotomy and translaryngeal jet ventilation. In: Roberts JR, Custalow CB, Thomsen TW, editors. Clinical procedures in emergency medicine. 4th edition. Philadelphia: Saunders; 2004. p. 120–33.
4. Brantigan CO, Grow JB Sr. Cricothyroidotomy: elective use in respiratory problems requiring tracheotomy. J Thorac Cardiovasc Surg 1976;71(1):72–81.
5. Hill C, Reardon R, Joing S, et al. Cricothyrotomy technique using gum elastic bougie is faster than standard technique: a study of emergency medicine residents and medical students in an animal lab. Acad Emerg Med 2010;17(6): 666–9.
6. Schaumann N, Lorenz V, Schellongowski P, et al. Evaluation of Seldinger technique emergency cricothyroidotomy versus standard surgical cricothyroidotomy in 200 cadavers. Anesthesiology 2005;102(1):7–11.
7. Holmes JF, Panacek EA, Sakles JC, et al. Comparison of 2 cricothyrotomy techniques: standard method versus rapid 4-step technique. Ann Emerg Med 1998; 32(4):442–6.
8. Chan TC, Vilke GM, Bramwell KJ, et al. Comparison of wire-guided cricothyrotomy versus standard surgical cricothyrotomy technique. J Emerg Med 1999; 17(6):957–62.
9. Benkhadra M, Lenfant F, Nemetz W, et al. A comparison of two emergency cricothyroidotomy kits in human cadavers. Anesth Analg 2008;106(1):182–5 Table of contents.
10. Schober P, Hegemann MC, Schwarte LA, et al. Emergency cricothyrotomy-a comparative study of different techniques in human cadavers. Resuscitation 2009;80(2):204–9.

11. DeLaurier GA, Hawkins ML, Treat RC, et al. Acute airway management. Role of cricothyroidotomy. Am Surg 1990;56(1):12–5.
12. Salvino CK, Dries D, Gamelli R, et al. Emergency cricothyroidotomy in trauma victims. J Trauma 1993;34(4):503–5.
13. Patel RG. Percutaneous transtracheal jet ventilation: a safe, quick, and temporary way to provide oxygenation and ventilation when conventional methods are unsuccessful. Chest 1999;116(6):1689–94.
14. Ezri T, Szmuk P, Warters RD, et al. Difficult airway management practice patterns among anesthesiologists practicing in the United States: have we made any progress? J Clin Anesth 2003;15(6):418–22.
15. McGill J, Clinton JE, Ruiz E. Cricothyrotomy in the emergency department. Ann Emerg Med 1982;11(7):361–4.
16. Erlandson MJ, Clinton JE, Ruiz E, et al. Cricothyrotomy in the emergency department revisited. J Emerg Med 1989;7(2):115–8.
17. Spaite DW, Joseph M. Prehospital cricothyrotomy: an investigation of indications, technique, complications, and patient outcome. Ann Emerg Med 1990;19(3):279–85.
18. Gillespie MB, Eisele DW. Outcomes of emergency surgical airway procedures in a hospital-wide setting. Laryngoscope 1999;109(11):1766–9.
19. Brantigan CO, Grow JB Sr. Subglottic stenosis after cricothyroidotomy. Surgery 1982;91(2):217–21.
20. Bair AE, Panacek EA, Wisner DH, et al. Cricothyrotomy: a 5-year experience at one institution. J Emerg Med 2003;24(2):151–6.
21. Shelden CH, Pudenz RH, Freshwater DB, et al. A new method for tracheotomy. J Neurosurg 1955;12(4):428–31.
22. Smith VM. Perforation of trachea during tracheotomy performed with Sheldon tracheotome. J Am Med Assoc 1957;165(16):2074–6.
23. Hamilton RD. Fatal hemorrhage during tracheotomy. Report of a case and use of Shelden tracheotome. JAMA 1960;174:530–1.
24. Toye FJ, Weinstein JD. A percutaneous tracheostomy device. Surgery 1969; 65(2):384–9.
25. Ciaglia P, Firsching R, Syniec C. Elective percutaneous dilatational tracheostomy. A new simple bedside procedure; preliminary report. Chest 1985;87(6):715–9.
26. Petros S. Percutaneous tracheostomy. Crit Care 1999;3(2):R5–10.
27. Byhahn C, Wilke HJ, Halbig S, et al. Percutaneous tracheostomy: Ciaglia Blue Rhino versus the basic Ciaglia technique of percutaneous dilational tracheostomy. Anesth Analg 2000;91(4):882–6.
28. Johnson JL, Cheatham ML, Sagraves SG, et al. Percutaneous dilational tracheostomy: a comparison of single- versus multiple-dilator techniques. Crit Care Med 2001;29(6):1251–4.
29. Kost KM. Endoscopic percutaneous dilatational tracheotomy: a prospective evaluation of 500 consecutive cases. Laryngoscope 2005;115(10 Pt 2):1–30.
30. Cianchi G, Zagli G, Bonizzoli M, et al. Comparison between single-step and balloon dilatational tracheostomy in intensive care unit: a single-centre, randomized controlled study. Br J Anaesth 2010;104(6):728–32.
31. Griggs WM, Worthley LI, Gilligan JE, et al. A simple percutaneous tracheostomy technique. Surg Gynecol Obstet 1990;170(6):543–5.
32. Anon JM, Gomez V, Escuela MP, et al. Percutaneous tracheostomy: comparison of Ciaglia and Griggs techniques. Crit Care 2000;4(2):124–8.
33. Kaiser E, Cantais E, Goutorbe P, et al. Prospective randomized comparison of progressive dilational vs forceps dilational percutaneous tracheostomy. Anaesth Intensive Care 2006;34(1):51–4.

34. Ambesh SP, Pandey CK, Srivastava S, et al. Percutaneous tracheostomy with single dilatation technique: a prospective, randomized comparison of Ciaglia blue rhino versus Griggs' guidewire dilating forceps. Anesth Analg 2002;95(6): 1739–45 Table of contents.

35. Anon JM, Escuela MP, Gomez V, et al. Percutaneous tracheostomy: Ciaglia Blue Rhino versus Griggs' guide wire dilating forceps. A prospective randomized trial. Acta Anaesthesiol Scand 2004;48(4):451–6.

36. Fikkers BG, Staatsen M, van den Hoogen FJ, et al. Early and late outcome after single step dilatational tracheostomy versus the guide wire dilating forceps technique: a prospective randomized clinical trial. Intensive Care Med 2011;37(7): 1103–9.

37. Karvandian K, Yousefian M, Khan ZH, et al. Comparative clinical trial between Ciaglia and Griggs techniques during tracheostomy performed in patients admitted to intensive care unit. Acta Med Iran 2012;50(8):525–9.

38. Kumar M, Trikha A, Chandralekha. Percutaneous dilatational tracheostomy: Griggs guide wire dilating forceps technique versus ULTRA-perc single-stage dilator - A prospective randomized study. Indian J Crit Care Med 2012;16(2):87–92.

39. Cabrini L, Landoni G, Greco M, et al. Single dilator vs guide wire dilating forceps tracheostomy: a meta-analysis of randomised trials. Acta Anaesthesiol Scand 2014;58(2):135–42.

40. Moller MG, Slaikeu JD, Bonelli P, et al. Early tracheostomy versus late tracheostomy in the surgical intensive care unit. Am J Surg 2005;189(3):293–6.

41. Griffiths J, Barber VS, Morgan L, et al. Systematic review and meta-analysis of studies of the timing of tracheostomy in adult patients undergoing artificial ventilation. BMJ 2005;330(7502):1243.

42. Heffner JE. Timing of tracheotomy in mechanically ventilated patients. Am Rev Respir Dis 1993;147(3):768–71.

43. Rumbak MJ, Newton M, Truncale T, et al. A prospective, randomized, study comparing early percutaneous dilational tracheotomy to prolonged translaryngeal intubation (delayed tracheotomy) in critically ill medical patients. Crit Care Med 2004;32(8):1689–94.

44. Terragni PP, Antonelli M, Fumagalli R, et al. Early vs late tracheotomy for prevention of pneumonia in mechanically ventilated adult ICU patients: a randomized controlled trial. JAMA 2010;303(15):1483–9.

45. Young D, Harrison DA, Cuthbertson BH, et al. Effect of early vs late tracheostomy placement on survival in patients receiving mechanical ventilation: the TracMan randomized trial. JAMA 2013;309(20):2121–9.

46. Ahmed N, Kuo YH. Early versus late tracheostomy in patients with severe traumatic head injury. Surg Infect (Larchmt) 2007;8(3):343–7.

47. Arabi Y, Haddad S, Shirawi N, et al. Early tracheostomy in intensive care trauma patients improves resource utilization: a cohort study and literature review. Crit Care 2004;8(5):R347–52.

48. Davidson SB, Blostein PA, Walsh J, et al. Percutaneous tracheostomy: a new approach to the emergency airway. J Trauma Acute Care Surg 2012;73(2 Suppl 1):S83–8.

49. Grant CA, Dempsey G, Harrison J, et al. Tracheo-innominate artery fistula after percutaneous tracheostomy: three case reports and a clinical review. Br J Anaesth 2006;96(1):127–31.

50. Lin JC, Maley RH Jr, Landreneau RJ. Extensive posterior-lateral tracheal laceration complicating percutaneous dilational tracheostomy. Ann Thorac Surg 2000; 70(4).1194 C.

51. Kedjanyi WK, Gupta D. Near total transection of the trachea following percutaneous dilatational tracheostomy. J R Coll Surg Edinb 2001;46(4):242–3.
52. Kornblith LZ, Burlew CC, Moore EE, et al. One thousand bedside percutaneous tracheostomies in the surgical intensive care unit: time to change the gold standard. J Am Coll Surg 2011;212(2):163–70.
53. Dennis BM, Eckert MJ, Gunter OL, et al. Safety of bedside percutaneous tracheostomy in the critically ill: evaluation of more than 3,000 procedures. J Am Coll Surg 2013;216(4):858–65 [discussion: 865–7].
54. Fikkers BG, van Veen JA, Kooloos JG, et al. Emphysema and pneumothorax after percutaneous tracheostomy: case reports and an anatomic study. Chest 2004; 125(5):1805–14.
55. Atkins JP. Current utilization of tracheotomy as a therapeutic measure. A review of the literature and an analysis of 526 cases. Laryngoscope 1960; 70:1672–90.
56. Francois B, Clavel M, Desachy A, et al. Complications of tracheostomy performed in the ICU: subthyroid tracheostomy vs surgical cricothyroidotomy. Chest 2003; 123(1):151–8.
57. Dillon JK, Christensen B, Fairbanks T, et al. The emergent surgical airway: cricothyrotomy vs tracheotomy. Int J Oral Maxillofac Surg 2013;42(2):204–8.
58. Freeman BD, Isabella K, Lin N, et al. A meta-analysis of prospective trials comparing percutaneous and surgical tracheostomy in critically ill patients. Chest 2000;118(5):1412–8.
59. Delaney A, Bagshaw SM, Nalos M. Percutaneous dilatational tracheostomy versus surgical tracheostomy in critically ill patients: a systematic review and meta-analysis. Crit Care 2006;10(2):R55.
60. Higgins KM, Punthakee X. Meta-analysis comparison of open versus percutaneous tracheostomy. Laryngoscope 2007;117(3):447–54.
61. Dulguerov P, Gysin C, Perneger TV, et al. Percutaneous or surgical tracheostomy: a meta-analysis. Crit Care Med 1999;27(8):1617–25.
62. Freeman BD, Isabella K, Cobb JP, et al. A prospective, randomized study comparing percutaneous with surgical tracheostomy in critically ill patients. Crit Care Med 2001;29(5):926–30.
63. Cobean R, Beals M, Moss C, et al. Percutaneous dilatational tracheostomy. A safe, cost-effective bedside procedure. Arch Surg 1996;131(3):265–71.

Integration of a Difficult Airway Response Team into a Hospital Emergency Response System

Monika Chmielewska, DO[a], Bradford D. Winters, PhD, MD[b],
Vinciya Pandian, PhD[c], Alexander T. Hillel, MD[a],*

KEYWORDS

- Difficult airway response team • Multidisciplinary • Difficult airway patient
- Rapid response system • Medical emergency teams • Rapid response teams

KEY POINTS

- Specialized equipment must be readily available during difficult airway responses and customized to specialty departments of the rapid-response system teams.
- The otolaryngologist contributes both nonsurgical techniques, such as rigid and flexible endoscopy, and surgical techniques that provide a valuable addition to a difficult airway response team.
- The collaboration between the Anesthesiology, Otolaryngology—Head and Neck Surgery, General Surgery, and Emergency Medicine departments includes highly experienced personnel with unique skills in securing a difficult airway.

INTRODUCTION

Hospital emergency response teams have evolved and expanded dramatically during the last couple of decades to provide acute care services well beyond the code team that traditionally responded to cardiopulmonary arrests.[1–3] Some of these teams are highly specialized focusing on specific disease states, such as, for myocardial infarction, the heart attack team (HAT) or, for strokes, the brain attack team (BAT). Others, such as the physician-led medical emergency team (MET) and the nurse-led rapid

We have no financial or funding sources to disclose.

[a] Department of Otolaryngology - Head and Neck Surgery, Johns Hopkins Hospital, 601 North Caroline Street, 6th Floor, Baltimore, MD 21287-0910, USA; [b] Department of Anesthesiology and Critical Care Medicine, Johns Hopkins Hospital, 1800 Orleans Street, Zayed 9127, Baltimore, MD 21287, USA; [c] Department of Anesthesiology and Critical Care Medicine, Johns Hopkins Hospital, 1800 Orleans Street, Phipps 409, Baltimore, MD 21287, USA

* Corresponding author.

E-mail address: ahillel@jhmi.edu

Anesthesiology Clin 33 (2015) 369–379

http://dx.doi.org/10.1016/j.anclin.2015.02.008
anesthesiology.theclinics.com

response team (RRT), address more general problems and respond to any deteriorating patient regardless of the disease process driving the deterioration.

Although there has been controversy regarding the effectiveness of this strategy, the accumulating evidence finds the MET-RRT intervention to be at least a moderately effective patient safety strategy. Reductions in the incidence of cardiopulmonary arrest and probable reductions in hospital mortality have been seen.[4–6] Its implementation has become nearly universal in Australian, Canadian, United States, and United Kingdom hospitals, as well as common in many other countries. Although there remain many questions regarding how to best implement MET-RRT programs and how to best optimize the afferent and efferent limb, as well as many others, this safety strategy is likely to remain and become as much the standard of care as cardiac arrest or code teams.[4,5]

The International Society for Rapid Response Systems, which grew out of the MET-RRT movement, has proposed that the panoply of emergency response teams that could exist within a hospital be described under the umbrella of a rapid-response system (RRS) that addresses all patient emergencies. A hospital's RRS could include a MET, an RRT, a BAT, a HAT, a code team, a massive transfusion team, and/or a difficult airway response team (DART) as well as any other teams the institution deems appropriate for their patient population. In some hospitals with more restricted resources, many of these teams may overlap. Regardless of how the hospital implements such a system, it is crucial to have clear processes and protocols for activating the correct team for the circumstance.

Although many of these types of emergency teams have become more ubiquitous, the DART remains perhaps less common than the others.[7] This may be a function of the greater number of publications regarding the MET-RRT strategy compared with the DART or because of the influence of drivers such as the Institute for Healthcare Innovation's 100K and 5 Million Lives campaigns,[8] and the Joint Commission's Patient Safety Goal #16.[9] Regardless of the reason, the DART approach and its treatment algorithms are particularly important to the overall RRS because a difficult airway may be encountered in any one of these scenarios. Patients are routinely intubated during cardiopulmonary arrests. Reports in the literature demonstrate that most MET-RRT activations are either specifically for respiratory distress (tachypnea, desaturation, dyspnea, or bradypnea) or on arrival to the patient bedside the team finds respiratory distress is a major part of the clinical scenario, requiring noninvasive or invasive ventilatory support.[10–28] Code teams and MET-RRTs are likely to encounter patients with difficult airways and need to know how to activate a DART response, if available, or have the ability to summon the appropriate expertise, absent a structured DART. If the hospital does have a structured DART program, the other teams that make up the RRS should be empowered and comfortable in activating it as soon as the situation requires airway control or any type of invasive mechanical ventilation.

A DART program was implemented at Johns Hopkins Hospital in 2008 in response to a consensus opinion that a more comprehensive management of the difficult airway is needed in patients outside of the operating room. DART was implemented with the goal of establishing a centralized response from airway experts and mobilizing specialized equipment used to secure the airway to the patient's bedside in the setting of a difficult airway. This article describes the DART program at Hopkins: how it is organized, what services contribute to it, and how it integrates into hospital management of the difficult airway patients outside of the operating room. DART was implemented with the goal of establishing a centralized response for at-risk patients and depicts systems put in place for management of difficult airway patients.

MULTIDISCIPLINARY TEAM

The Hopkins DART Program has led to improved outcomes for the last 7 years and it is a successful multidisciplinary model to highlight. It is a collaborative effort between 4 departments: Anesthesiology and Critical Care Medicine, General Surgery, Otolaryngology—Head and Neck Surgery, and Emergency Medicine (when the difficult airway occurs in the emergency department). The DART team responds to active difficult airway situations on the hospital inpatient floor, in the emergency department, intensive care unit (ICU), procedural area, and the operating rooms suite. The 3 core components of the program are operations, safety, and education. The operations component includes responding team members, establishment of a universal paging system, a standardized DART cart, and real-time documentation of management of the difficult airway patients. The safety component reports all DART events into an electronic airway registry, conducts in situ simulations, and manages quarterly morbidity and mortality conferences with the 4 departments present. The goal is rapid feedback to the team based on past airway events, thus improving future responses. Finally, the education aspect of DART organizes a difficult airway management course for fellows and senior residents. The education seminars focus on teaching skills that are necessary in the difficult airway setting via hands-on stations, as well as team-building exercises. The interaction between multiple specialties builds familiarity and trust that carries over when responding to a difficult airway event in the hospital.[29]

It is known that effective teamwork, communication, and coordination among health care providers can aid in preventing adverse patient outcomes.[30] As a result, in recent years there has been a new hospital focus on the multidisciplinary approach to the difficult airway patient. Grant Medical Center in Ohio, a level-one trauma center, established a response team for events of impending respiratory compromise. This involved only simulated cases with a future goal of incorporating the new policies to improve patient care. The DART is comprised of anesthesiologists, trauma surgeons, anesthesia aide, primary nurse, respiratory therapist, and pharmacist. An educational program was devised that included didactic and skill testing using computerized patient simulators and self-paced observations. Results showed significant improvement in the knowledge of managing a difficult airway comparing the pretest results to the 30-days after education results.[7]

Flavin and colleagues[31] implemented a multidisciplinary team approach to the airway management of their ICU patients. This intervention concentrated on the presence of key airway equipment, education of team members, and the accompaniment of senior anesthesiologists for intubations. Analysis of endotracheal intubations before and after this intervention demonstrated a decrease in reintubation rates and a decrease in attempts at initial intubation.

EQUIPMENT

Standardized equipment carts are a critical component of the DART operations. Carts are strategically located around the hospital for proximity to high utility floors or ICUs and are mobilized to the bedside once a DART is activated. Airway equipment and supplies considered to be efficacious and often used for difficult airway patients have been made available on the cart. Each DART cart includes 2 sizes of fiberoptic bronchoscopes, a rigid bronchoscope, rigid laryngoscopes (Dedo and Holinger), a cricothyrotomy set, a tracheostomy set, and laryngeal mask airways (**Fig. 1**). Maintenance of these carts includes an inventory checklist that is completed by a nurse and equipment manager every time the cart is used. Additionally, weekly checks of the

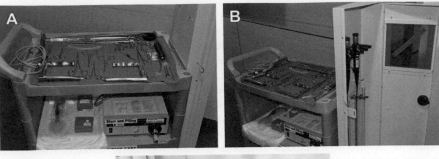

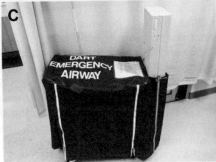

Fig. 1. DART cart. (*A, B*) The equipment found on the DART cart. (*C*) Standard cover on the DART cart.

equipment on the carts occur to ensure proper working order. Hospitals may consider a narrower set of equipment and airway techniques depending on the team members who will make up their DART.

INDICATIONS AND PROCESS

The indications for DART activation at Hopkins include patients with a history of difficult airway who need imminent intubation and patients who pose difficulty in securing the airway during a code response. A flow chart depicting the response process used to activate the DART is shown in **Fig. 2**. Data analyzing DART responses from July 2008 to June 2013 showed that the most common activations occurred in the ICU (53%) followed by the ward (22%) and the emergency room department (18%). Fifty-four percent of DART calls occurred between 7 AM and 7 PM. Although the goal is complete team presence at the patient's bedside within 10 minutes, the database from the last 5 years shows a mean response time of 6 minutes.

Ideally, the DART should use the same activation steps as the MET-RRT or code teams, given the immediacy of the threat to the patient's life. Clearly, however, hospitals may elect to tailor their process. It is not expected that a critical access hospital have the same resources or capabilities as does a large tertiary academic teaching hospital. However, each should develop a standardized plan and process for how to respond to such emergencies. If a special number is called for codes then that same number should be used for the DART with a clearly specified algorithm for team dispatchers to use in sending the appropriate teams, akin to the 911 universal activation. Having a different activation protocol for each type of team in the RRS (eg, call operator for the code team but directly page the DART) creates confusion for frontline providers and may result in dangerous delays in response times and the risk of not activating the correct team or not getting all members of the team.

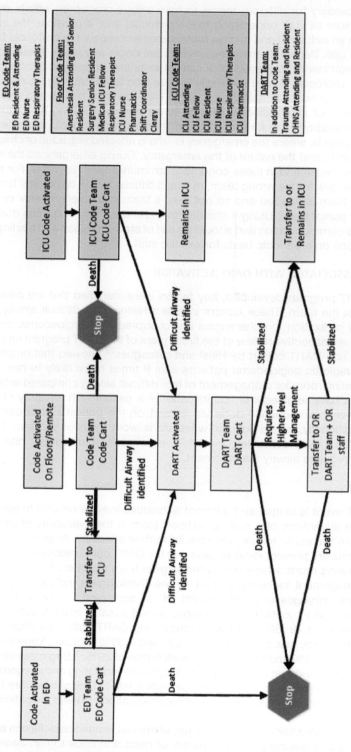

Fig. 2. DART response process. ED, emergency department; OHNS, otolaryngology—Head and neck surgery.

If it is necessary for different teams to have unique processes, efforts should be made to ensure all staff understand these protocols and, if possible, the institution should have an industrial and human factors engineer review the protocols for clarity and ease of use. Because emergency events can occur anywhere, these algorithms should be prominently displayed in all clinical areas and possibly in nonclinical areas as well. The protocols should minimally include who to contact (eg, operator, emergency room) and how (eg, telephone, page, Web-based). They should also provide guidance for what information to provide to the person receiving the request for a dispatch, preferably in the form of a script. The script should include elements such as who the caller is, where the emergency is, who is affected (eg, adult or child, patient or not a patient), and the nature of the emergency. During emergencies the stress on the staff is immense and in these conditions communication may falter. For example, the caller may ask for the wrong team, making it difficult for the dispatcher to ascertain which RRS team is needed and so not send a team in a timely manner or send an incorrect or partial team. Using a standardized approach and script can dramatically improve this communication and should be part of staff education and training for new staff and done on a periodic basis for existing staff.

FACTORS ASSOCIATED WITH DART ACTIVATION

As the DART program developed, key factors were identified that are crucial in the activation of the team. These factors include a history of a difficult airway, cervical spine injury or fixation, oropharyngeal and/or supraglottic angioedema, and airway bleeding. A retrospective review of the first 2 years of the DART program and comparison with a non-DART cohort by Hillel and colleagues[29] showed that oropharyngeal and/or supraglottic angioedema patients were 9 times more likely to require a visit to the operating room for management of their difficult airway compared with patients who did not have angioedema. Identification of a patient with a history of a known difficulty airway is frequently done via an alert on the patient's electronic medical record. Additionally, a blue hospital wristband is worn by these patients. Therefore, for any future airway difficulties, the DART response is automatically initiated when the patient requires airway management.

TECHNIQUES

Each DART event is unique and different techniques may be needed to establish the airway. The advantage of a multidepartment team is the availability of experienced staff that are trained in techniques specific to their specialty. Anesthesiologists and their residents are present in-house and lead the DART calls unless patients are taken to the operating room, where one of the surgical team members takes the lead. The airway management techniques used by anesthesiologists include Macintosh and Miller blade laryngoscopy, placement of a supraglottic airway followed by fiberoptic-guided intubation, and fiberoptic-guided nasal or oral intubation. Anesthesiologists secured 49 (60%) of the airways during DART calls from 2008 to 2010.[29] Blade laryngoscopy was the primary method used in 39% of cases, followed by videolaryngoscopy at 24% and fiberoptic nasal intubation at 20%.[29] Bag mask ventilation is another vital method that is used to keep the patient ventilating and oxygenated while the airway plan is devised. The anesthesiologist's role is critical to secure the airway and also for the administration of intravenous medications to keep the patient sedated and comfortable.

In a patient with a known medical history of trismus, limited neck flexion and extension, craniofacial disorders, macroglossia, or head and neck tumor, awake flexible endoscopically guided nasotracheal intubation can be attempted.[32] Contraindication to this technique includes skull base fractures.[33] Both anesthesiologists and otolaryngologists are trained in this technique. DART data over 2 years showed that anesthesiologists and the otolaryngology surgeon used fiberoptic nasal intubation successfully as their method of choice with the same frequency, 20% and 23% of the time, respectively. If time allows, the patient's nasal passage can be decongested with oxymetazoline nasal spray and anesthetized with lidocaine jelly on a nasal trumpet. The flexible fiberoptic bronchoscope with the endotracheal tube is passed transnasally with direct visualization of the larynx. The endoscope is introduced through the epiglottis into the subglottic area and the endotracheal tube is slid over the bronchoscope into the trachea.

The skill set of rigid laryngoscopy and increased knowledge about head and neck anatomy are unique to otolaryngology head and neck surgery. Through training and educational courses, residents become proficient in both flexible and rigid laryngoscopy, as well as surgical airways such as cricothyroidotomy and tracheostomy. Additionally, because otolaryngology residents are exposed to head and neck patients frequently, they become very familiar with head and neck anatomy. Otolaryngologists can play a vital role as part of a response team for the management of patients with difficult airway. In a cohort of 90 DART patients from 2008 to 2010, difficult airways were secured by an otolaryngologist 36% of the time.[29] The Holinger and Dedo laryngoscopes are routinely used during laryngology cases. The Holinger laryngoscope is especially useful in the setting of a difficult intubation because the tubed design helps navigate edematous tissue and the anterior flange improves access to the larynx. In the cohort of 90 patients, laryngoscopy was used 40% of the time by an otolaryngologist to secure the airway. According to Iseli and colleagues, the surgeon's familiarity with the anterior commissure scope (Holinger) and bougie was useful in airways that were anatomically distorted, actively bleeding, or had an obstructed view of the glottis. In this study, they found that superior intubation outcomes were seen with the team approach involving an anesthesiologist trained in head and neck and the head and neck surgeon.[34]

Patients with upper airway obstruction or massive hemoptysis pose a challenge in securing the airway secondary to decreased visualization of the larynx. Bronchoscopy can be an effective technique and vital skill set necessary for this patient population. Causes of upper airway obstruction include acute aspiration of a foreign body, trauma, inflammation, tumors, and stenosis. Massive hemoptysis is most commonly from a pulmonary source such as bronchiectasis or necrotizing pneumonia. Bronchoscopy has traditionally been performed in the operating room under general anesthesia or deep sedation; however, it is increasingly being performed outside of the operating room setting by interventional pulmonologists and thoracic surgeons.[35] Flexible bronchoscopy allows for suctioning secretions such as mucus or blood, thus improving visualization. Rigid bronchoscopy allows for instrumentation via the bronchoscope while oxygenating and ventilating using the side port or jet. Although this is not commonly used in the setting of the difficult airway patient and was performed only in 7% of patients in 2 years, it can be a life-saving skill for this patient population.[29]

In the setting of "cannot intubate, cannot ventilate," an emergency surgical airway is indicated. The skills of securing a surgical airway via cricothyrotomy are critical to have when endotracheal intubation has failed or is not an option. Cricothyrotomy is a technique that is most frequently performed by otolaryngologists and trauma surgeons; however, all physicians should be familiar with the procedure should they find themselves in an emergency situation without a more experienced surgeon present. The key landmarks include the inferior aspect of the thyroid cartilage and cricoid cartilage separated by the cricothyroid membrane. A vertical skin incision is made in the midline, the soft tissue quickly dissected off the cricothyroid membrane, which is punctured to enter the airway. Cricothyrotomy should be considered a temporary airway and the authors recommend converting to a tracheostomy within 72 hours to lessen the risk of injury to the vocal folds and subglottic stenosis at the level of the narrow cricoid.[36]

POSTPROCEDURE CARE

Education and training for the RRS process is critical.[37–41] However, although education is essential, it is known to be a relatively weak intervention to improve patient safety and quality when compared with interventions that use force functions and cognitive tools such as checklists.[42] Thus when the focus is on education and training it is understood that some forms of education and training are better than others and that the strongest forms of education available are needed to optimize its effect. Multimodal education using strategies best suited to adult learners are particularly effective, especially when simulation exercises are part of the educational process.[41] Whether these sessions are in a proper simulation laboratory or out on the general ward, they rely on engaging all of the senses and cognitive processes necessary for the real events; unlike slide presentations and examination questions, which tend to focus only on the knowledge components. Research shows that these multimodal types of learning activities result in improved performance. They should be used whenever possible.

The education and safety committees of DART have the common goal of improving future responses. For 7 years, 18 airway courses were organized for the fellows and residents. These courses were taught by experienced staff familiar with participating in the DART responses at Johns Hopkins. This training developed individual knowledge and skills in managing difficult airway patients, taught team-based approaches, and enhanced professional relationships between the staff and the residents and fellows.

The safety committee reports each DART event within 24 hours to an electronic Web-based registry developed by the Anesthesiology and Critical Care Medicine department. Obtaining and documenting the data allows retrospective review of the outcomes and creates improvements for future DART calls. The database keeps track of the general patient information and event details, specifically the participants in the event, and the techniques and equipment used to secure the airway. The data are promptly reviewed by the oversight committee and their suggestions shared. The committee is composed of the chairs, quality improvement physician-directors, and residency directors from each specialty. Additionally, cases are reviewed and discussed at quarterly morbidity and mortality conferences.

FUTURE CONSIDERATIONS/SUMMARY

Structured DARTs are not commonly part of the RRS in most hospitals and, therefore, cannot be considered the standard of care in the United States. The DART is complex both in terms of staffing and necessary equipment. It requires several layers of expertise (Anesthesiology, General Surgery, Otolaryngology—Head and Neck Surgery, and Emergency departments) as well as very expensive specialized equipment.[7] These resources may not be readily available at many hospitals part or all of the time. Therefore, defining what a DART should include and whether a hospital can meet any of those requirements on a part-time or full-time basis remains unclear. What is clear, however, is that any hospital can and likely will encounter a patient with a difficult airway in urgent or emergent conditions. Managing the difficult airway may become the responsibility of the code team and/or the MET-RRT. Even if a hospital cannot support a full-fledged DART program, such hospitals should develop contingency plans and protocols for how their non-DART RRS teams will manage a difficult airway situation when it presents.

A well-established hospital-wide DART has skilled personnel responding to difficult airways encountered outside the operating room setting. DART is an effective program that incorporates the Right People, Right Parts, and Right Place[7] approach in the safe management of the difficult airway. These acutely ill patients require prompt treatment and the DART model effectively mobilizes special equipment and skilled personnel to their bedside. Since 2008, the Johns Hopkins DART program represents a model to improve patient safety for the management of difficult airway patients. Although the resources used in this program may not be feasible for every hospital, implementation of some components could provide effective difficult airway patient care with available resources.

REFERENCES

1. DeVita MA, Bellomo R, Hillman K, et al. Findings of the first consensus conference on medical emergency teams. Crit Care Med 2006;34:2463–78.
2. Buist MD, Jarmolowski E, Burton PR, et al. Recognising clinical instability in hospital patients before cardiac arrest or unplanned admission to intensive care. A pilot study in a tertiary-care hospital. Med J Aust 1999;171:22–5.
3. Franklin C, Mathew J. Developing strategies to prevent in hospital cardiac arrest: analyzing responses of physicians and nurses in the hours before the event. Crit Care Med 1994;22:244–7.
4. Jones DA, DeVita MA, Bellomo R. Rapid-response teams. N Engl J Med 2011; 365:139–46.
5. Winters BD, Weaver SJ, Pfoh ER, et al. Rapid-response systems as a patient safety strategy a systematic review. Ann Intern Med 2013;158:417–25.
6. Chan PS, Jain R, Nallmothu BK, et al. Rapid response teams: a systematic review and meta-analysis. Arch Intern Med 2010;170:18–26.
7. Long L, Vanderhoff B, Smyke N, et al. Management of difficult airways using a hospital-wide "Alpha Team" approach. Am J Med Qual 2010;25(4):297–304.
8. Institute for Healthcare Improvement. 5 Million Lives Campaign: Overview. Available at: www.ihi.org/offerings/Initiatives/PastStrategic Initiatives/5MillionLivesCampaign/Pages/default.aspx on 1. Accessed November 8, 2014.
9. Joint Commission on Accreditation of Healthcare Organizations. 2008 National Patient Safety Goals. Jt Comm Perspect 2007;27:10–22.
10. Bristow PJ, Hillman KM, Chey T, et al. Rates of in-hospital arrests, deaths and intensive care admissions: the effect of a medical emergency team. Med J Aust 2000;173:236–40.
11. Buist MD, Moore GE, Bernard SA, et al. Effects of a medical emergency team on reduction of incidence of and mortality from unexpected cardiac arrests in hospital: preliminary study. BMJ 2002;324:387–90.
12. Bellomo R, Goldsmith D, Uchino S, et al. A prospective before-and-after trial of a medical emergency team. Med J Aust 2003;179:283–7.
13. DeVita MA, Braithwaite RS, Mahidhara R, et al. Medical Emergency Response Improvement Team (MERIT). Use of medical emergency team responses to reduce hospital cardiopulmonary arrests. Qual Saf Health Care 2004;13:251–4.
14. Kenward G, Castle N, Hodgetts T, et al. Evaluation of a medical emergency team one year after implementation. Resuscitation 2004;61:257–63.

15. Dacey MJ, Mirza ER, Wilcox V, et al. The effect of a rapid response team on major clinical outcome measures in a community hospital. Crit Care Med 2007;35:2076–82.
16. Baxter AD, Cardinal P, Hooper J, et al. Medical emergency teams at The Ottawa Hospital: the first two years. Can J Anaesth 2008;55:223–31.
17. Chan PS, Khalid A, Longmore LS, et al. Hospital-wide code rates and mortality before and after implementation of a rapid response team. JAMA 2008;300: 2506–13.
18. Medina-Rivera B, Campos-Santiago Z, Palacios AT, et al. The effect of the medical emergency team on unexpected cardiac arrest and death at the VA Caribbean Healthcare System: a retrospective study. Crit Care Shock 2010;13:98–105.
19. Rothberg MB, Belforti R, Fitzgerald J, et al. Four years' experience with a hospitalist-led medical emergency team: an interrupted time series. J Hosp Med 2012;7:98–103.
20. Offner PJ, Heit J, Roberts R. Implementation of a rapid response team decreases cardiac arrest outside of the intensive care unit. J Trauma 2007;62:1223–7.
21. Beitler JR, Link N, Bails DB, et al. Reduction in hospital wide mortality after implementation of a rapid response team: a long-term cohort study. Crit Care 2011;15: R269.
22. Hatler C, Mast D, Bedker D, et al. Implementing a rapid response team to decrease emergencies outside the ICU: one hospital's experience. Medsurg Nurs 2009;18:84–90, 126.
23. Konrad D, Jäderling G, Bell M, et al. Reducing in-hospital cardiac arrests and hospital mortality by introducing a medical emergency team. Intensive Care Med 2010;36:100–6.
24. Laurens N, Dwyer T. The impact of medical emergency teams on ICU admission rates, cardiopulmonary arrests and mortality in a regional hospital. Resuscitation 2011;82:707–12.
25. Lighthall GK, Parast LM, Rapoport L, et al. Introduction of a rapid response system at a United States veterans affairs hospital reduced cardiac arrests. Anesth Analg 2010;111:679–86.
26. Santamaria J, Tobin A, Holmes J. Changing cardiac arrest and hospital mortality rates through a medical emergency team takes time and constant review. Crit Care Med 2010;38:445–50.
27. Shah SK, Cardenas VJ Jr, Kuo YF, et al. Rapid response team in an academic institution: does it make a difference? Chest 2011;139:1361–7.
28. Tobin AE, Santamaria JD. Medical emergency teams are associated with reduced mortality across a major metropolitan health network after two years service: a retrospective study using government administrative data. Crit Care 2012;16:R210.
29. Hillel AT, Pandian V, Mark L, et al. A novel role for otolaryngologists in the multidisciplinary difficult airway response team. Laryngoscope 2015;125(3):640–4.
30. Mark LJ, Herzer KR, Akst S, et al. General considerations of anesthesia and management of the difficult airway. In: Flint PW, editor. Cummings otolaryngology-head & neck surgery. 5th edition. Philadelphia: Mosby; 2010. p. 108–20.
31. Flavin K, Horsnby J, Fawcett J, et al. Structured airway intervention improves safety of endotracheal intubation in an intensive care unit. Br J Hosp Med (Lond) 2012;73:341–4.
32. Vidya B, Cariappa KM, Kamath AT. Current perspectives in intra operative airway management in maxillofacial trauma. J Maxillofac Oral Surg 2012;11(2):138–43.
33. Iseli T, Iseli C, Golden B, et al. Outcomes of intubation in difficult airways to head and neck pathology. Ear Nose Throat J 2012;91(3):E1–5.

34. Worrell S, DeMeester S. Thoracic emergencies. Surg Clin North Am 2014;94: 183–91.
35. Jose R, Shaefi S, Navani N. Anesthesia for bronchoscopy. Curr Opin Anaesthesiol 2014;27:453–7.
36. Patel S, Meyer T. Surgical airway. Int J Crit Illn Inj Sci 2014;4(1):71–6.
37. Buist M, Bellomo R. MET: the emergency medical team or the medical education team? Crit Care Resusc 2004;6:88–91.
38. Jones D, Baldwin I, McIntyre T, et al. Nurses' attitudes to a medical emergency team service in a teaching hospital. Qual Saf Health Care 2006;15:427–32.
39. Bagshaw SM, Mondor EE, Scouten C, et al. A survey of nurses' beliefs about the medical emergency team system in a Canadian tertiary hospital. Am J Crit Care 2010;19:74–83.
40. DeVita MA, Hillman K. Potential sociological and political barriers to medical emergency team implementation. In: DeVita MA, Hillman K, Bellomo R, editors. Medical emergency teams: implementation and outcome measurement. New York: Springer Science and Business Media; 2006. p. 91–103.
41. DeVita MA, Schaefer J, Lutz J, et al. Improving medical emergency team (MET) performance using a novel curriculum and a computerized human patient simulator. Qual Saf Health Care 2005;14:326–31.
42. Winters BD, Gurses AP, Lehmann H, et al. Clinical review: checklists - translating evidence into practice. Crit Care 2009;13(6):210.

Preparedness and Education in Airway Management

Paul Baker, MBChB, MD, FANZCA

KEYWORDS

- Airway management • Education • Simulation
- Competency-based medical education • Simulation-based medical education
- Deliberate practice • Simulation-based mastery learning

KEY POINTS

- Inadequate education and training are major factors contributing to patient morbidity and mortality in airway management.
- Preemptive thinking and planning are essential components of safe airway management.
- Simulation-based medical education (SBME) has efficacy similar to that of traditional medical education.
- Deliberate practice is a more effective indicator of expertise than experience or academic achievement.

PREPAREDNESS AND EDUCATION

The purpose of medical education at all levels is to prepare physicians with knowledge, skills, and features of professionalism needed to deliver quality patient care.[1]

Traditional Medical Education

Most anesthesiologists have honed their skills in the operating room during many hours of clinical practice; this is the traditional method of medical education that

Disclosure: Dr P. Baker has received airway management equipment for teaching and research purposes from a number of companies including Olympus, Karl Storz, Covidien, LMA, Ambu, Parker, Welch Allyn, Cook, King Systems, Verathon, and Truphatek. He also owns Airway Simulation Limited, which manufactures the ORSIM bronchoscopy simulator.
Department of Anaesthesiology, University of Auckland, Level 12, Room 081, Auckland Support Building 599, Park Road, Grafton, Private Bag 92019, Auckland 1142, New Zealand
E-mail address: paul@airwayskills.co.nz

Anesthesiology Clin 33 (2015) 381–395
http://dx.doi.org/10.1016/j.anclin.2015.02.007
1932-2275/15/$ – see front matter © 2015 Elsevier Inc. All rights reserved.

anesthesiology.theclinics.com

was formalized into an apprenticeship model by William Halsted more than 100 years ago. Learning depends on exposure to clinical cases of varying difficulty and can be improved by supervision and teaching. This method of experiential learning has advantages of managing real anatomy, physiology, and pathology in a stream of variety and complexity. Experience is conveniently gained during working hours without absence from operating sessions to attend lectures or workshops. The apprenticeship model remains the most common form of medical education and has supporters who argue that competency-based medical education (CBME) is too prescriptive, thereby missing the broader qualities of being a physician.[2] It is also claimed that CBME tends to dwell on mere competence and therefore sets a low standard for readiness to practice and tends to be top-down, applying primarily to trainees.[3]

Despite this support, the traditional medical education model has the following flaws[4]:

1. Clinical exposure to complex patients is serendipitous, and therefore the development of airway experience is proportional to working hours. The type of case mix, increasing use of alternative airway devices such as supraglottic airways (SGAs), regional anesthesia, and clinical placement can all adversely affect airway skill development. Some technical skills develop slowly because of the low incidence of difficult airways (**Table 1**). One study concluded that up to 200 endotracheal intubations, under supervision, may be required before trainee anesthesiology residents achieve a 95% success rate in the operating room.[5] A similar study examined the learning curve for the laryngeal mask airway in first year anesthesiology residents and found that supervision was deemed necessary for the first 40 insertions.[6]

2. With traditional medical education, patients are inevitably exposed to novices; this has direct implications on patient safety, particularly with high-risk procedures required for airway management. Novice bronchoscopists have an increased complication rate during the first trimester of their bronchoscopy training, which can influence the success rate of positive biopsy results.[11,12] Direct laryngoscopy and tracheal intubation have a success rate of only 50% in novices, with a heightened risk of esophageal intubation during this time.[13]

3. Teaching airway management in the operating room is not ideal, because it can increase the workload of the instructing anesthesiologist and cause distraction from patient care.[14] Ethical issues arise if patients are used for training purposes when the airway procedures are either unnecessary or unsafe.[15–18]

4. Airway equipment is often introduced into departments with little training or reference to instructions.[19] Practitioners are often self-taught or are taught by

Table 1
Gaining experience at managing complex airway problems inevitably takes time because of the low incidence of difficult airways

Difficult intubation	6.2%[7]
Difficult bag mask ventilation	1.4%[8]
Difficult bag mask ventilation, difficult laryngoscopy	0.4%[7]
Impossible bag mask ventilation	0.15%[9]
Impossible laryngeal mask	1.1%[10]
Impossible intubation, difficult bag mask ventilation	0.3%[7]
Impossible intubation, impossible ventilation	0.0019%[9]

Data from Refs.[7–10]

colleagues and use devices without any formal instruction.[20] This practice has led to morbidity such as oral trauma caused by tracheal tube stylets during video laryngoscopy.[21] Failure to read the instructions and incorrect use of equipment have also led to fatal outcomes with airway exchange catheters.[22]

These problems call for a reexamination of the current practice of education in airway management. Other options are available to complement traditional clinical experience.

Simulation-Based Medical Education

Simulation offers several advantages, particularly given the problems associated with traditional airway management training in the operating room (**Box 1**).

Issenberg and colleagues[23] have listed desirable features that make simulators preferable to traditional educational models, namely, validity, feedback, repetitive practice, curriculum integration, varying levels of difficulty, multiple learning strategies, capturing clinical variation, controlled environment, individualized learning, and defined outcomes or benchmarks. Unfortunately, this comprehensive list of features is not incorporated in many forms of skills training.

Simulation provides the learner opportunities to improve knowledge, skill, and behavior in a safe and controlled environment. According to Gaba,[24] "Simulation is a technique - not a technology – to replace or amplify real experiences with guided experiences that evoke or replicate substantial aspects of the real world in a fully interactive manner." SBME uses "devices, trained persons, lifelike virtual environments and contrived social situations that mimic problems, events, or conditions that arise in professional encounters."[23] Extensive research, including meta-analyses, studying the efficacy of this form of education confirms the benefits of SBME in comparison with no treatment and traditional clinical education.[1,25]

Mastery Learning

Mastery learning is a strict form of CBME in which the learner is required to meet predetermined goals before progressing to the next instructional objective. The aim of mastery learning is for learners to achieve a consistent standard and complete all educational goals, irrespective of the time required to reach those goals. At least 7 complementary features have been described for mastery learning (**Box 2**).

Cook and colleagues[26] published a meta-analysis and systematic review of mastery learning for health professionals, using technology-enhanced simulation. Results showed that mastery SBME was associated with large effects on skills and moderate effects on patient outcomes.

Box 1
Advantages of simulation

1. Training is conducted without patient involvement
2. Mistakes can occur repeatedly without harm
3. Performance can be recorded and assessed for future feedback
4. Procedures can be easily interrupted for feedback
5. Exposure to difficult and unusual scenarios can be created and rehearsed regularly
6. Trainees can learn at their own rate

Box 2
The 7 complementary features for mastery learning

1. Baseline or diagnostic assessment

2. Clear learning objectives sequenced as units of increasing difficulty

3. Engagement in powerful and sustained educational activities (eg, deliberate skills practice, data interpretation, reading) focused on reaching objectives

4. A fixed minimum passing standard (eg, test score, checklist percentage)

5. Formative assessment with specific feedback to gauge unit completion at the minimum passing standard for mastery

6. Advancement to the next educational unit given measured achievement at or above the mastery standard (summative assessment)

7. Continued practice or study on an educational unit until the mastery standard is reached

From McGaghie WC, Issenberg SB, Barsuk JH, et al. A critical review of simulation-based mastery learning with translational outcomes. Med Educ 2014;48:376; with permission.

Translational Outcomes

Translational outcomes concern the implications of education beyond the teaching environment. These implications include cost savings, skill retention, and improved patient outcomes. The face value of some simulators can be high, but cost saving may be significant. Expensive repairs for flexible bronchoscopes can be reduced by up to 84% by training on simulators.[27] Skill retention, technical ability, and compliance with an algorithm for cricothyroidotomy for up to 1 year were enhanced by simulation training.[28] A systematic review of the literature suggests that simulation-based training is as effective as traditional patient-based training for colonoscopy, endoscopic sinus surgery, and laparoscopic camera navigation.[29]

e-Learning

e-Learning is the use of Internet technology to enhance knowledge. A wide range of applications for Web-based information include online libraries for research, Internet repositories for course notes, interactive learning with feedback and assessment, case-based learning, hypermedia, and simulations. Content can be delivered synchronously with real-time, instructor-led e-learning (teleconferencing, Internet chat forums, and instant written or visual messaging). Alternatively, content can be delivered asynchronously, where delivery and receipt of information is not simultaneous. The instructor and learner can communicate by e-mail, bulletin boards, or Weblogs, but not in real time. Using e-learning can potentially free educators from their roles as resources of information to facilitators of learning and assessment. Research concerning effectiveness of e-learning suggests that results are equivalent to those of traditional lecture-based learning.[30]

Social Media Medical Education

The volume of new literature appearing daily is increasing exponentially. It is almost impossible to keep up with current knowledge through publication. Using free open access medical education, which includes blogs, podcasts, microblogs (such as Twitter), and smartphone apps, readers can rely on feeds about relevant articles and join in chat groups to share ideas. Using this medium, information is disseminated and discussed instantly and globally, long before conventional journal publications.

The significant downside of this form of medical education is the lack of robust review processes. A common ground has been suggested whereby journals could operate their own blog sites moderated by clinicians, and publications could be discussed, reviewed, and corrected online.[31]

Confidence Versus Competence

Education in airway management is not limited to trainees. Senior practitioners also need training to maintain skills, particularly with new devices. Without regular practice, skills can deteriorate, and this is aggravated by advancing years whereby psychomotor skills decline after 45 years of age.[32] Self-awareness of declining ability by senior practitioners is poor. Typically, they overrate their ability, and this tendency increases with age.[33] The impact of overconfidence is also evident in teaching. Residents, who tend to overrate their knowledge, are often cast in the role as teachers of medical students. These are 2 examples of the Kruger-Dunning effect, which explain the inverse relationship of competence and confidence.[34] In these examples, the more one learns, the less confident one becomes with the realization of one's limitations.

An Airway Management Curriculum

Curriculum review is underway with many organizations involved in medical education. The Australian and New Zealand College of Anaesthetists (ANZCA) have recently adopted a new CBME curriculum that includes airway management as a clinical fundamental. For trainees, a graduated program incorporates specific objectives that must be achieved and performance that must be demonstrated at each stage. For specialists, a revised CBME program has been implemented, which includes 4 clinical fundamentals to be completed each triennium. These fundamentals include anaphylaxis, cardiopulmonary resuscitation, massive transfusion, and "cannot intubate, cannot oxygenate."

The adoption of airway management into the new CBME curriculum will increase the demand for airway management training. This trend has been evident for several years in North America with a growing number of residency programs in the United States and Canada. Ideally, the following certain criteria should apply:

1. A systematic and graduated approach to build on previous knowledge and skills (**Box 3**).
2. A syllabus based on current guidelines and best practice (**Box 4**).
3. Use of various educational options including e-learning, didactic instruction, simulation-based medical education (SBME), clinical instruction, and self-directed learning.
4. Opportunity for the trainee to engage in practice with immediate feedback and the chance to repeat performance with modified behavior.
5. Assessment to ensure competency at each level before advancement.
6. Instructors overseeing these programs should have skills in medical education and advanced knowledge in airway management.

Practice Guidelines

Airway management guidelines form a foundation for airway education provided they are current and based on a systematic review of good evidence; this is particularly important if the guidelines are to be used medicolegally for standards of practice.[35] Guidelines can be a source for cognitive aids that help improve performance. Cognitive aids are prompts, mnemonics, charts, and graphics designed to improve performance and patient outcome during anesthetic emergencies, such as the management of malignant

---

Box 3
An example of a minimal skill set to be acquired by a trainee during an airway rotation

- Optimal bag mask ventilation technique.
- Optimal direct laryngoscopy and intubation with a range of laryngoscopes and intubation aids.
- The use of supraglottic airways.
- The use of rigid optical devices including video laryngoscopes and optical stylets.
- The use of flexible bronchoscopes.
- Cricothyroidotomy.

From Baker PA, Weller JM, Greenland KM, et al. Education in airway management. Anaesthesia 2011;66:103; with permission.

---

hyperthermia.[36] A recent meta-analysis of simulation studies examining technical performance found that the majority observed an improvement in performance after the use of cognitive aids.[37] Important features of cognitive aids include their content, design, utilization during training, and inclusion during team building.[37] These aids invariably draw on information from practice guidelines and can be used in real time. An example of a cognitive aid for airway management is the Vortex approach (**Fig. 1**).[38] In contrast to a cognitive aid, practice guidelines contain more detail, are based on literature and peer

---

Box 4
Items that might be included in an airway management program

- Airway anatomy and physiology.
- Assessment of the airway.
- The maintenance of oxygenation and ventilation.
- Avoidance of trauma during airway management.
- Utilization of preplanned strategies.
- The importance of calling for help and when to do this.
- Airway algorithms.
- Management of known and unexpected difficult airways.
- Establishment and confirmation of an open airway.
- Awake intubation.
- Rapid sequence induction.
- Intubation via a supraglottic airway
- Retrograde intubation.
- Emergency techniques for cannot-ventilate cannot-oxygenate situations.
- Extubation strategies.
- Dissemination of information concerning the critical airway.
- Human factor training in relation to airway management.

From Baker PA, Weller JM, Greenland KM, et al. Education in airway management. Anaesthesia 2011;66:104; with permission.

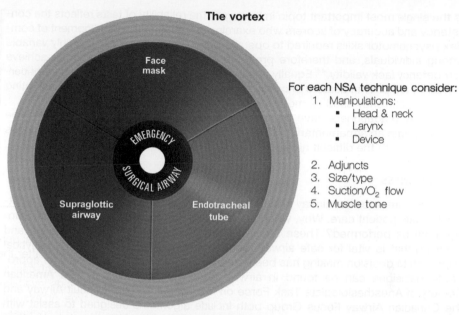

The vortex

Face mask

EMERGENCY SURGICAL AIRWAY

Supraglottic airway

Endotracheal tube

For each NSA technique consider:
1. Manipulations:
   - Head & neck
   - Larynx
   - Device

2. Adjuncts
3. Size/type
4. Suction/O_2 flow
5. Muscle tone

Maximum 3 tries at each nonsurgical airway technique
At least 1 try should be had by the most experienced available clinician

Fig. 1. The Vortex approach. A cognitive aid for airway management. (*Courtesy of* Nicholas Chrimes, MBChB, FANZCA and Peter Fritz, MBChB, FACEM, Melbourne, Australia.)

review, and can take time to assimilate, limiting their use during an emergency when practitioners struggle to remember lists and are prone to fixation error.

Human Factors

Knowledge and skill need to be supplemented by an understanding of human factors in providing safe airway management. Common human factor themes have been found to contribute or cause significant errors that lead to patient morbidity and mortality in airway management.[39] Poor communication and teamwork, system errors with failure to check, individual failings such as fixation error, inadequate leadership, poor situation awareness, and fatigue are recurring themes.

Specific courses that incorporate human factor and teamwork training are now compulsory components of training for continuing professional development by the ANZCA. The Effective Management of Anesthetic Crises course includes a half day dedicated to airway crises and includes skills stations, airway drills, and instruction on human error and decision making.[40]

A systematic review of a small number of studies recently examined the translation of crisis resource management (CRM) skills acquired in simulation training. Results suggest that CRM skills are transferred to the workplace and that these skills may contribute to improved patient outcomes including decreased mortality.[41]

Assessment

Implicit in the CBME model is the concept that each competency should be teachable, learnable, and measurable.[42] Assessment is therefore an integral part of modern education, and assessments require proof of validity and reliability. Validation establishes the ability of a test to measure what it is supposed to measure and is regarded as the single most important topic in testing.[43] The reliability of tests reflects the consistency and accuracy of scorers who examine those tests. The development of complex psychomotor skills required to operate a flexible bronchoscope is highly variable among individuals, and therefore predetermined number of procedures to achieve competency lack validity.[44] Equally, the use of log books and self-assessment of performance are poor indicators of competence.[45] Validated checklists and global rating scales are currently used as more reliable forms of assessment.[46]

If airway practitioners have been well prepared through education, they will be equipped with an armamentarium when confronted with the decisions and challenges associated with the difficult airway.

PREPAREDNESS

Education prepares the airway practitioner for important decisions, which can be critical for safe patient care. Why, where, how, when, and by whom should airway management be performed? These questions are part of the preemptive thinking and planning that is vital for safe airway management, and a structured and analytical approach to decision making has been proposed.[47] Information necessary for appropriate decisions can be found in airway management guidelines. The American Society of Anesthesiologists Task Force on Management of the Difficult Airway and the Canadian Airway Focus Group both include algorithms designed to assist with decision making.[48–50] Serious morbidity and mortality can arise when these matters are overlooked. The Fourth National Audit Project (NAP4) of the Royal College of Anaesthetists and the Difficult Airway Society identified poor judgment as the second most common causal and contributory factor (59%) after patient factors (77%).[39] The ability to make informed decisions comes not only from experience but also from a lifelong commitment to medical education and learning.

Why

Before embarking on a prescribed airway plan, consider whether airway management is necessary. Some airway procedures are performed wherein simple alternatives would be preferable, such as sedation or local anesthesia. If airway difficulty occurs unexpectedly, a wise decision is to wake the patient up, rather than persevering with potentially traumatic intubation attempts.

Where

Decide whether appropriate equipment, expertise, assistance, and backup are available in the current environment. In a hospital where a patient's airway is a concern, it might be prudent to secure the airway in the operating room before off-the-floor procedures. Conversely, a decision to transfer before airway management requires careful consideration of the risks involved during transport. Some circumstances unavoidably dictate suboptimal locations for airway management, such as off-the-floor, out-of-hospital, and battlefield situations. Despite this, highly trained retrieval teams of physicians can achieve impressive success rates of intubation and cricothyroidotomy before transport.[51] Safe airway management in the field before transfer can also be assisted by telebation, using telecommunication technology to link a less-experienced practitioner to an expert during airway management.[52]

How

A wide range of airway techniques and devices are available to manage the airway. Deciding which is the most appropriate depends on the skill and experience of the practitioner and the context of the airway management.[53] Equipment needs to be fit for purpose and comply with a minimum standard of evidence.[54,55] Devices can be tailored to fit the patient's anatomy with the objective of "matching the right device with the right patient in the hands of a practitioner with the right skills."[56,57]

If bag mask ventilation, SGA, or tracheal intubation look to be difficult, a comprehensive airway plan should be implemented. Alternative plans should be discussed with the team, including an elective awake oral, nasal, or surgical airway. An awake technique may not be feasible if the patient is uncooperative, has copious secretions or an occluding upper airway lesion, declines consent, or has local anesthetic reactions. Choice between rapid sequence induction or inhalation induction will depend on the risk of aspiration. If an awake procedure is not possible, preoperative identification of the cricothyroid membrane with ultrasonography, placement of a cricothyroid cannula, and a double set-up in preparation for an emergency cricothyroidotomy is possible. It is also wise to involve an experienced surgeon who can rapidly perform an emergency surgical airway, should the need arise. In the NAP4 study, surgeons performing surgical airways achieved a 100% success rate, including 11 cases of failed cannula cricothyroidotomies performed by anesthetists.[39]

When

The timing of airway intervention depends on the urgency and clinical presentation of the patient. A partially obstructed airway caused by angioneurotic edema or laryngotracheobronchitis could improve with medical treatment, thereby avoiding the need for instrumentation of the airway. In contrast, early intubation is indicated in a patient with airway burns who might otherwise steadily deteriorate toward total airway obstruction. Fasting protocols should be followed to ensure gastric emptying if the urgency of the procedure permits.

By Whom

A patient with a known difficult airway should be managed by the most skillful person available. A child with a congenital airway anomaly, for example, ideally requires care from an experienced pediatric team, familiar with pediatric airways and including a pediatric anesthesiologist and pediatric otorhinolaryngologist. Skill and experience, combined with careful selection of equipment and techniques, help avoid multiple intubation attempts, airway obstruction, and cardiovascular complications. Trained assistants are vital members of airway management teams, and their presence has been shown to improve safety during a simulated anesthesiology crisis.[58] A preoperative team briefing helps assistants understand their role in the airway management plan. For an emergency induction of anesthesia, multiple staff might be required, in which case, clear allocation of roles should be defined. To assist tracheal intubation, particularly in the intensive care unit or emergency department, an emergency induction checklist can be followed.[59] Use of a checklist reduces the number of missing items required to induce anesthesia (**Fig. 2**).[60] Even when all these contingencies are in place, however, it is wise to plan for failure. Evidence shows that only half of the patients with a difficult airway are anticipated preoperatively.[61,62]

WHAT IS COMPETENCE AND EXPERTISE

Competence defines the minimum capability required to perform a task. The terms competent, proficient, and expert describe a spectrum of skill development, and each of these terms should be used in the context of the difficulty of the task and the educational goal. Competence at managing a normal airway, for example, is

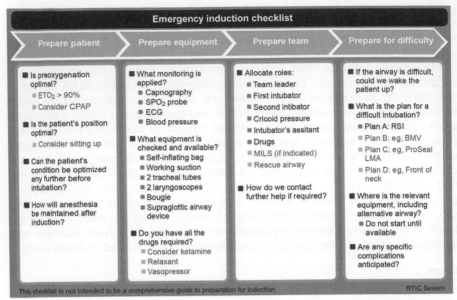

Fig. 2. A checklist for use before emergency department intubation. BMV, Bag mask ventilation; CPAP, Continuous Positive Airway Pressure; ECG, Electrocardiograph; ETO$_2$, End tidal oxygen; LMA, Laryngeal mask airway; MILS, Manual in-line stabilisation; RSI, Rapid sequence induction; SPO$_2$, Saturation of peripheral oxygen. (*Courtesy of* The Royal College of Anaesthetists, London, United Kingdom.)

not equivalent to competence at managing a difficult airway. This concept is important when defining the educational goal and selecting simulators for airway management training. Simple part-task trainers are appropriate for novices who aim to achieve competence on normal airways but do not replicate the reality of a difficult airway. Reducing the reality gap between simulation and the clinical environment increases the transfer of learning.[63] Overtraining on the same part-task trainers does not help expert learners who are trying to move up the learning curves of more advanced procedures and retain that skill. Expert learners benefit from higher-fidelity training.[64,65]

Anesthesiologists cannot necessarily assume the title of airway experts based on their years of medical practice. Long experience decreases the effort of performance and makes it automatic, but it does not increase the quality of performance.[66] From research on individuals engaged in sport and music, Ericsson has identified characteristic behaviors typical of experts: deliberate practice, with immediate feedback; problem solving; evaluation; and the opportunity to modify and repeat performance. These form the building blocks for expert performance. Deliberate practice drives learners to more challenging experiences, thereby continuously pushing them to the limit of their ability and beyond. One characteristic of an expert is the ability to adapt to unusual challenging situations. In the context of airway management, an expert practitioner is able to choose from a range of techniques and devices to suit the patient. This versatility can only be achieved by deliberate practice and distributed learning over a long period. In the model proposed by Ericsson,[67] initial learning tends to be rapid because individuals move through the cognitive and associative phases and eventually reach automaticity wherein procedures are performed with little effort (**Fig. 3**). The danger of automaticity is that improvement can become arrested so that individuals

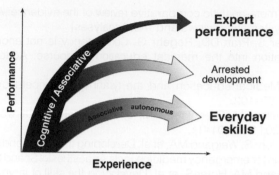

Fig. 3. Illustration of the qualitative difference between the course of improvement of expert performance and of everyday activities. The goal for everyday activities is to reach as rapidly as possible a satisfactory level that is stable and autonomous. After individuals pass through the cognitive and associative phases, they can generate their performances virtually automatically with a minimal amount of effort (see the gray/white plateau at the bottom of the graph). In contrast, expert performers counteract automaticity by developing increasingly complex mental representations to attain higher levels of control of their performance and will, therefore, remain within the cognitive and associative phases. Some experts will at some point in their career give up their commitment to seeking excellence and thus terminate regular engagement in deliberate practice to further improve performance, which results in premature automation of their performance. (*From* Ericsson KA. Deliberate practice and acquisition of expert performance: a general overview. Acad Emerg Med 2008;15:988–94; with permission.)

have difficulty modifying their behavior to cope with a challenging and unusual situation. Evidence suggests that deliberate practice is a more effective indicator of expertise than experience or academic achievement.[68]

Although certain comfort can be gained from repeatedly using the same airway device to intubate every patient, such as the size 3 Macintosh laryngoscope, the inevitable failure rate will require an alternative device on some occasions. Airway practitioners need to be equally adept with alternative devices, to cope with such unexpected presentations.

Changes in practice over the past 10 years indicate an increasing use of video laryngoscopes, bougies and SGAs, with declining use of flexible bronchoscopy and direct laryngoscopy.[69] Under these circumstances, skill decay can only be avoided by purposeful deliberate practice with devices such as the flexible bronchoscope. Adoption of a new device such as the video laryngoscope involves learning. A 7-year study of video laryngoscope use in an institution showed improvement of first-pass intubation success in that time.[70]

SUMMARY

The goal of medical education is to create well-rounded practitioners who are equipped with the skills, knowledge, and behavior to safely manage patients with difficult airways. With the expertise gained from this education, appropriate decisions that will decrease patient morbidity and mortality can be made.

REFERENCES

1. McGaghie WC, Issenberg SB, Cohen ER, et al. Does simulation-based medical education with deliberate practice yield better results than traditional clinical

education? A meta-analytic comparative review of the evidence. Acad Med 2011; 86:706–11 [systematic reviews and meta-analyses].

2. Jarvis-Selinger S, Pratt DD, Regehr G. Competency is not enough: integrating identity formation into the medical education discourse. Acad Med 2012;87: 1185–90.

3. Brooks MA. Medical education and the tyranny of competency. Perspect Biol Med 2009;52:90–102.

4. Baker PA, Weller JM, Greenland KM, et al. Education in airway management. Anaesthesia 2011;66:101–11.

5. Bernhard M, Mohr S, Weigand MA, et al. Developing the skill of endotracheal intubation: implication for emergency medicine. Acta Anaesthesiol Scand 2012;56:164–71.

6. Mohr S, Weigand MA, Hofer S, et al. Developing the skill of laryngeal mask insertion: prospective single center study. Anaesthesist 2013;62:447–52.

7. Langeron O, Cuvillon P, Ibanez-Esteve C, et al. Prediction of difficult tracheal intubation: time for a paradigm change. Anesthesiology 2012;117:1223–33.

8. Kheterpal S, Han R, Tremper KK, et al. Incidence and predictors of difficult and impossible mask ventilation. Anesthesiology 2006;105:885–91.

9. Kheterpal S, Martin L, Shanks AM, et al. Prediction and outcomes of impossible mask ventilation: a review of 50,000 anesthetics. Anesthesiology 2009;110:891–7 [systematic reviews and meta-analyses].

10. Ramachandran SK, Mathis MR, Tremper KK, et al. Predictors and clinical outcomes from failed laryngeal mask airway Unique™: a study of 15,795 patients. Anesthesiology 2012;116:1217–26 [systematic reviews and meta-analyses].

11. Ouellette DR. The safety of bronchoscopy in a pulmonary fellowship program. Chest 2006;130:1185–90.

12. Knight RK, Clarke SW. An analysis of the first 300 fibreoptic bronchoscopies at the Brompton Hospital. Br J Dis Chest 1979;73:113–20.

13. Mulcaster JT, Mills J, Hung OR, et al. Laryngoscopic intubation: learning and performance. Anesthesiology 2003;98:23–7.

14. Weinger MB, Reddy SB, Slagle JM. Multiple measures of anesthesia workload during teaching and nonteaching cases. Anesth Analg 2004;98:1419–25 [table of contents].

15. Cook TM. Intubation training in the real world. Anaesthesia 2008;63:434–6 [author reply: 436–8].

16. Cormack RS, Lehane JR. Intubation training in the real world: a defence of the Northwick Park drill. Anaesthesia 2007;62:975–8.

17. Goldberg JS, Bernard AC, Marks RJ, et al. Simulation technique for difficult intubation: teaching tool or new hazard? J Clin Anesth 1990;2:21–6.

18. Wheeler DW, Williams CE, Merry AF. Pulling the plug on ad hoc critical incident training. Br J Anaesth 2009;103:145–7.

19. Brain AI. The last resort–follow the instructions! Anaesthesia 1999;54:116.

20. Dawson AJ, Marsland C, Baker P, et al. Fibreoptic intubation skills among anaesthetists in New Zealand. Anaesth Intensive Care 2005;33:777–83.

21. Cooper RM. Complications associated with the use of the GlideScope videolaryngoscope. Can J Anaesth 2007;54:54–7.

22. Duggan LV, Law JA, Murphy MF. Brief review: supplementing oxygen through an airway exchange catheter: efficacy, complications, and recommendations. Can J Anaesth 2011;58:560–8.

23. Issenberg SB, McGaghie WC, Petrusa ER, et al. Features and uses of high-fidelity medical simulations that lead to effective learning: a BEME systematic review. Med Teach 2005;27:10–28 [systematic reviews and meta-analyses].

24. Gaba DM. The future vision of simulation in health care. Qual Saf Health Care 2004;13(Suppl 1):i2–10.
25. Cook DA, Hatala R, Brydges R, et al. Technology-enhanced simulation for health professions education: a systematic review and meta-analysis. JAMA 2011;306:978–88 [systematic reviews and meta-analyses].
26. Cook DA, Brydges R, Zendejas B, et al. Mastery learning for health professionals using technology-enhanced simulation: a systematic review and meta-analysis. Acad Med 2013;88:1178–86 [systematic reviews and meta-analyses].
27. Lunn W, Garland R, Gryniuk L, et al. Reducing maintenance and repair costs in an interventional pulmonology program. Chest 2005;127:1382–7.
28. Hubert V, Duwat A, Deransy R, et al. Effect of simulation training on compliance with difficult airway management algorithms, technical ability, and skills retention for emergency cricothyrotomy. Anesthesiology 2014;120:999–1008 [systematic reviews and meta-analyses].
29. Dawe SR, Pena GN, Windsor JA, et al. Systematic review of skills transfer after surgical simulation-based training. Br J Surg 2014;101:1063–76 [systematic reviews and meta-analyses].
30. Ruiz JG, Mintzer MJ, Leipzig RM. The impact of E-learning in medical education. Acad Med 2006;81:207–12.
31. Weingart SD, Faust JS. Future evolution of traditional journals and social media medical education. Emerg Med Australas 2014;26:62–6.
32. Siu LW, Boet S, Borges BC, et al. High-fidelity simulation demonstrates the influence of anesthesiologists' age and years from residency on emergency cricothyroidotomy skills. Anesth Analg 2010;111:955–60.
33. Choudhry NK, Fletcher RH, Soumerai SB. Systematic review: the relationship between clinical experience and quality of health care. Ann Intern Med 2005;142:260–73 [systematic reviews and meta-analyses].
34. Kruger J, Dunning D. Unskilled and unaware of it: how difficulties in recognizing one's own incompetence lead to inflated self-assessments. J Pers Soc Psychol 1999;77:1121–34.
35. Crosby ET. An evidence-based approach to airway management: is there a role for clinical practice guidelines? Anaesthesia 2011;66(Suppl 2):112–8.
36. Harrison TK, Manser T, Howard SK, et al. Use of cognitive aids in a simulated anesthetic crisis. Anesth Analg 2006;103:551–6.
37. Marshall S. The use of cognitive aids during emergencies in anesthesia: a review of the literature. Anesth Analg 2013;117:1162–71.
38. Sillen A. Cognitive tool for dealing with unexpected difficult airway. Br J Anaesth 2014;112:773–4.
39. Cook TM, Woodall N, Frerk C. Major complications of airway management in the UK: results of the Fourth National Audit Project of the Royal College of Anaesthetists and the Difficult Airway Society. Part 1: anaesthesia. Br J Anaesth 2011;106:617–31 [systematic reviews and meta-analyses].
40. Weller J, Morris R, Watterson L, et al. Effective Management of Anaesthetic Crises: development and evaluation of a college-accredited simulation-based course for anaesthesia education in Australia and New Zealand. Simul Healthc 2006;1:209–14.
41. Boet S, Bould MD, Fung L, et al. Transfer of learning and patient outcome in simulated crisis resource management: a systematic review. Can J Anaesth 2014;61:571–82 [systematic reviews and meta-analyses].
42. Brasel KJ, Bragg D, Simpson DE, et al. Meeting the Accreditation Council for Graduate Medical Education competencies using established residency training program assessment tools. Am J Surg 2004;188:9–12.

43. Downing SM, Haladyna TM. Validity and its threats. In: Downing SM, editor. Assessment in health professions education. New York: Routledge; 2009. p. 21–55.
44. Pastis NJ, Nietert PJ, Silvestri GA. American College of Chest Physicians Interventional chest/diagnostic procedures network steering C: variation in training for interventional pulmonary procedures among US pulmonary/critical care fellowships: a survey of fellowship directors. Chest 2005;127:1614–21.
45. Bould MD, Crabtree NA. Are logbooks of training in anaesthesia a valuable exercise? Br J Hosp Med (Lond) 2008;69:236.
46. Bould MD, Crabtree NA, Naik VN. Assessment of procedural skills in anaesthesia. Br J Anaesth 2009;103:472–83.
47. Yentis SM. Decision analysis in anaesthesia: a tool for developing and analysing clinical management plans. Anaesthesia 2006;61:651–8.
48. Practice Guidelines for Management of the Difficult Airway. An updated report by the American Society of Anesthesiologists Task Force on Management of the Difficult Airway. Anesthesiology 2013;118:251–70 [systematic reviews and meta-analyses].
49. Law AJ, Broemling N, Cooper RM, et al. The difficult airway with recommendations for management-Part 1-Difficult tracheal intubation encountered in an unconscious/induced patient. Can J Anaesth 2013;60:1089–118 [systematic reviews and meta-analyses].
50. Law AJ, Broemling N, Cooper RM, et al. The difficult airway with recommendations for management-Part 2-The anticipated difficult airway. Can J Anaesth 2013;60:1119–38 [systematic reviews and meta-analyses].
51. Lockey D, Crewdson K, Weaver A, et al. Observational study of the success rates of intubation and failed intubation airway rescue techniques in 7256 attempted intubations of trauma patients by pre-hospital physicians. Br J Anaesth 2014;113:220–5.
52. Mosier J, Joseph B, Sakles JC. Telebation: next-generation telemedicine in remote airway management using current wireless technologies. Telemed J E Health 2013;19:95–8.
53. Hung O, Murphy M. Context-sensitive airway management. Anesth Analg 2010;110:982–3.
54. Baker PA, Flanagan BT, Greenland KB, et al. Equipment to manage a difficult airway during anaesthesia. Anaesth Intensive Care 2011;39:16–34.
55. Pandit JJ, Popat MT, Cook TM, et al. The Difficult Airway Society 'ADEPT' guidance on selecting airway devices: the basis of a strategy for equipment evaluation. Anaesthesia 2011;66:726–37.
56. Greenland KB, Irwin MG. Airway management–'spinning silk from cocoons' (-Chinese idiom). Anaesthesia 2014;69:296–300.
57. Kristensen MS, Teoh WH, Asai T. Which supraglottic airway will serve my patient best? Anaesthesia 2014;69:1189–92.
58. Weller JM, Merry AF, Robinson BJ, et al. The impact of trained assistance on error rates in anaesthesia: a simulation-based randomised controlled trial. Anaesthesia 2009;64:126–30.
59. Cook T, Behringer EC, Benger J. Airway management outside the operating room: hazardous and incompletely studied. Curr Opin Anaesthesiol 2012;25:461–9.
60. Thomassen O, Storesund A, Softeland E, et al. The effects of safety checklists in medicine: a systematic review. Acta Anaesthesiol Scand 2014;58:5–18.
61. Baker PA, Moore CL, Hopley L, et al. How do anaesthetists in New Zealand disseminate critical airway information? Anaesth Intensive Care 2013;41:334–41.

62. Pearce A, Shaw J. Airway assessment and planning, NAP4. In: Cook T, Woodall N, Frerk CM, editors. Major complications of airway management in the United Kingdom. London: The Royal College of Anaesthetists and the Difficult Airway Society; 2011. p. 135–42.
63. Grierson LE. Information processing, specificity of practice, and the transfer of learning: considerations for reconsidering fidelity. Adv Health Sci Educ Theory Pract 2014;19:281–9.
64. Kolozsvari NO, Kaneva P, Brace C, et al. Mastery versus the standard proficiency target for basic laparoscopic skill training: effect on skill transfer and retention. Surg Endosc 2011;25:2063–70.
65. Aggarwal R, Mytton OT, Derbrew M, et al. Training and simulation for patient safety. Qual Saf Health Care 2010;19(Suppl 2):i34–43.
66. Ericsson KA. Expertise. Curr Biol 2014;24:R508–10.
67. Ericsson KA. Deliberate practice and acquisition of expert performance: a general overview. Acad Emerg Med 2008;15:988–94.
68. Ericsson KA. The influence of experience and deliberate practice on the development of superior expert performance. In: Ericcson KA, Charness N, Feltovich PJ, et al, editors. The Cambridge Handbook of Expertise and Expert Performance. New York: Cambridge University Press; 2006. p. 683–703.
69. Wanderer JP, Ehrenfeld JM, Sandberg WS, et al. The changing scope of difficult airway management. Can J Anaesth 2013;60:1022–4.
70. Sakles JC, Mosier J, Patanwala AE, et al. Improvement in GlideScope Video Laryngoscopy performance over a seven-year period in an academic emergency department. Intern Emerg Med 2014;9:789–94.

What We All Should Know About Our Patient's Airway

Difficult Airway Communications, Database Registries, and Reporting Systems Registries

Jessica Feinleib, MD, PhD[a],*, Lorraine Foley, MD, MBA[b], Lynette Mark, MD[c]

KEYWORDS

- Difficult airway letter • Airway documentation • Patient notification
- Airway registries • Airway databases • Hospital information systems
- MedicAlert national difficult airway/intubation registry

KEY POINTS

- The American Society of Anesthesiologists, Canadian Airway Focus Group Difficult Airway Society, the Society for Airway Management, and other international airway societies recommend the following steps for disseminating difficult airway information: (1) a written report or letter for the patient, (2) a report to the medical record, (3) a chart flag, (4) communication with the patient's surgeon or primary caregiver, and (5) a notification bracelet or equivalent identification device.
- Institutions would be well served to create in-house difficult airway alerts, standardized airway documentation, airway registries, and "Dear Patient" difficult airway letters.
- Hospital policies regarding sedation and out-of-operating room intubation and extubation should be adapted to include safeguards for patients with documented difficult airways.

INTRODUCTION

All airway practitioners encounter a difficult airway, and likely encounter a failed airway, during their career. The consequences of failed airway maintenance and endotracheal intubation are devastating to the patient, the practitioner, and the health care system.[1] Complex airway management is a multifaceted problem involving health care providers in a variety of clinical settings. Although a large percentage of difficult intubations can be predicted via a careful review of history and airway examination,

[a] Yale University School of Medicine, New Haven CT, 333 Cedar Street, New Haven, CT 06510, USA; [b] Winchester Hospital, Tufts School of Medicine, 41 Highland Avenue, Boston, MA 01890, USA; [c] Johns Hopkins University School of Medicine, 1800 Orleans Street, ZB 6214, Baltimore, MD 21287, USA
* Corresponding author.
E-mail address: jessica@feinleib.md

Anesthesiology Clin 33 (2015) 397–413
http://dx.doi.org/10.1016/j.anclin.2015.02.010
1932-2275/15/$ – see front matter Published by Elsevier Inc.
anesthesiology.theclinics.com

unanticipated difficult airways are still reported at a rate of 1% to 3% among hospitalized operative patients.[2–5] Since Cooper's classic 1978 paper on human errors, anesthesiology has made great strides to reduce preventable harm.[6] A history of a difficult airway and its recognition as a risk factor for future airway management has been helpful in the mitigation of risk in the clinical management of the difficult airway patient.[7,8] Additionally, technology and new devices have improved anesthesiologists' ability to secure airways. Remaining difficulties include the cryptic anatomy encounter or other anatomic barriers to airway maintenance that were not communicated. Thus, a new "human error" of airway safety is poor forward information transmission. The critical data lacking often include identification of such patients along with the complete documentation of airway management techniques that failed and those that were successful. The effective and efficient dissemination of this critical airway information to health care providers and patients is the current task set to our interdisciplinary professions.

Whereas the patient's difficult airway was most likely first made evident in the setting of an operating room, subsequent events could occur in a variety of settings (even in the home or in public places) and involve physician or nonphysician providers, such as paramedics, emergency room physicians, physicians of other specialties (eg, otolaryngology), certified registered nurse anesthetists, and/or anesthesiologists. Therefore, it is incumbent on airway physicians to make every effort to identify difficult airway patients in and out of the operating room and transmit this knowledge in widely accessible forms using terminology that is directed toward other airway specialists, health care providers, and patients or laypersons. The fundamental differences between the successful management of known versus unanticipated difficult airways are clearly seen in the enhanced patient outcomes observed in the former scenario.[2,9,10]

Currently, numerous difficult airway communication reporting mechanisms exist, including airway databases and registries, although the field is migrating from a nascent stage toward a more nationally and internationally integrated stage. This transition is nonetheless still characterized by many competing elements, fractured systems, and diverse goals. We present a taxonomy of difficult airway databases, registries, and clinical practices that have been successfully implemented.

CURRENT DIFFICULT AIRWAY DATABASES
Systems in Place

There are two major goals of difficult airway databases: to identify specific patients for their protection and to improve their future care; and to collect data to learn about the epidemiology and cause of difficult airways to improve systems of care and clinical practice. Based on these goals, there are three types of difficult airway databases: (1) patient protective difficult airway database; (2) epidemiologic and etiologic difficult airway database; and (3) combined patient protective, epidemiologic, and etiologic difficult airway database. The first two accomplish one, but not both of the aforementioned goals as would be the ideal (**Fig. 1**). Other important features include the time frame (either time limited or perpetual) and accessibility for data reporting and retrieval. Data reporting can be restricted to predetermined institutions and patients or may be broadened to include global data reporting and retrieval. The data elements that are collected obviously determine the use of that databank. For incidence and prevalence calculations, the denominator of the total number of airway management occurrences is needed and the numerator of untoward airway events. To illustrate this taxonomy of difficult airway database, we have reviewed and analyzed multiple examples, highlighting their strengths and weaknesses. The databases are grouped

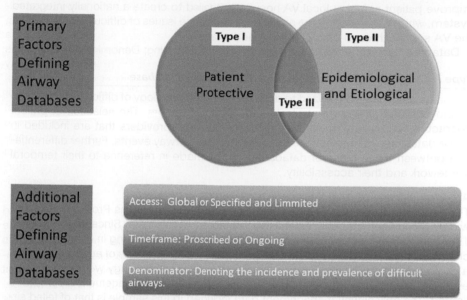

Fig. 1. Taxonomy of difficult airway databases.

according to the criteria depicted in **Fig. 1** and at the end of each synopsis, any additional factors defining that airway database are encapsulated. This discussion is not an exhaustive listing of all difficult airway databases, but covers the most substantial ones. This analysis also provides a framework for the evaluation of such databases and guidance for future discussions about difficult airway database goals and their future use.

Type I: Patient Protective Difficult Airway Database

These databases are organized to identify and protect individual patients during their hospitalization and for their future care. It has long been the practice of many anesthesiology groups to keep an informal record of patients with difficult airways. Many groups have over time gone on to formalize this collective knowledge into more comprehensive databases, patient record flags, and patient notification systems. These databases are usually limited to a specific location or anesthesiology practice and access to this information is usually confined to that group.

Veterans Affairs Healthcare System

In 2012 the Veterans Affairs (VA) Healthcare System (approximately 150 hospitals) set forth a comprehensive series of airway management standards through the Out of Operating Room Airway Management directive (VHA Directive 2012-032). Included in this series of standards were guidelines stating that all VA hospitals had to have "a plan for managing the known or emergently identified difficult airway" and "a process for notifying such patients." The implementation method of these guidelines was left to the individual VA hospitals to determine. Most VA hospitals now have a difficult airway patient electronic flag; however, these flags are only local VA flags and do not attach to the patient's national electronic record. The establishment of a national patient record flag requires congressional assent. Additionally, the airway information collected by each VA hospital is not standardized, nor is there a searchable database of the information collected across the VA system. Although this directive sought to improve patient safety at local VA hospitals, it failed to create a nationally integrated system, which has impeded the ability to ascertain the issues of difficult airways within the VA system through data collection and analysis.

Database Factors: Access, Limited; Timeframe, Ongoing; Denominator, None.

Type II: Epidemiologic and Etiologic Difficult Airway Database

These databases are organized to determine the epidemiology of difficult airways or to catalog difficult airway events to identify etiologic factors. The selection of patient characteristics, airway management techniques, and providers that are included in these databases determines their use for analyzing airway events. Further differentiation between these types of databases can be made in reference to their temporal framework and their accessibility.

American Society of Anesthesiologists Closed Claims Project

The American Society of Anesthesiologists (ASA) Closed Claims Project is the most widely recognized and fully established database of this type. Since its inception in 1984, this group has analyzed anesthesia-related events resulting in completed legal claims in the United States.[9] The results of these multiple rounds of analysis have had a profound and positive impact on the practice of anesthesiology worldwide.[9] However, the usefulness of these data in the context of airway management is somewhat limited. The only airway management data included in this sample is that of failed airways that produced morbidity and mortality, and that by definition resulted in a legal contest. Such bias to the most extreme airway events lacks the inclusion of a total number of airway management attempts needed to determine an event incidence. Moreover, because these data are based on insurance claims, rich clinical detail may be lacking.

Database Factors: Access, Limited; Timeframe, Ongoing; Denominator, None.

National Emergency Airway Registry and National Emergency Airway Registry for children

The National Emergency Airway Registry (NEAR) is an ongoing project established in 2003. It prospectively collects emergency department intubation data from more than 30 international institutions (http://www.near.edu/index.cfm). This World Wide Web–based database includes more than 16,000 emergency department intubations defined by a standardized data collection form. The data are only accessible to the participating institutions for analysis and publication of findings, and are deidentified. As such, this registry is incapable of providing providers and patients with airway information for future airway management. However, this database collects information on all intubations, regardless of difficulty, allowing for the calculation of incidence and prevalence of airway factors within the population of participating institutions.

NEAR for children (NEAR4KIDS) was established subsequently to NEAR and further focuses on pediatric intensive care unit intubation data. (http://www.near.edu/near4kids/welcome.cfm). It was originally comprised of a handful of institutions and has now grown to include 22 children's hospitals.

Database Factors: Access, Limited; Timeframe, Ongoing; Denominator, Included.

National Audit Project 4

The National Audit Project 4 (NAP-4) was a time-limited joint effort of the Difficult Airway Society and the Royal College of Anaesthetists. Over a 1-year period (September 2008–September 2009) all participating UK hospitals documented every airway management event that resulted in an unanticipated intensive care unit admission, death, brain damage, or an emergency surgical airway (http://www.das. uk.com/nataauditproject).[10] These data were then carefully analyzed for patient and provider factors that precipitated these events. In addition the event rates could be calculated because of the inclusion of all airway management occurrences in the database system. This audit resulted in a profound reexamination of airway management outside of the operating room and during extubation. However, the data collection time frame was limited and therefore only provides a snapshot view of airway events. Determination of any change in airway management event rate subsequent to this period requires an additional audit.

Database Factors: Access, Limited; Timeframe, Proscribed; Denominator, Calculated.

Australia and New Zealand Emergency Department Airway Registry

In response to the results of the NAP-4 effort, the Australia and New Zealand Emergency Department Airway Registry was established by emergency physicians in 2011 (http://www.airwayregistry.org.au/registry.html). It prospectively collects data from all intubations preformed in approximately 20 emergency departments in Australia and New Zealand. This registry's data are submitted by a clinical champion at each site via a standardized and patient deidentified form. The inclusion of all airway management occurrences in the database system allows for the calculation of airway morbidity and mortality rates. Since NAP-4, multiple national databases, similar to this one, have been enacted (Danish system; https://clinicaltrials.gov/show/NCT01718561).

Database Factors: Access, Limited; Timeframe, Ongoing; Denominator, Included.

Anesthesia Quality Institute: Anesthesia Incident Reporting System

The Anesthesia Incident Reporting System collects data on all anesthesia incidents, including those relating to airway management events. These data are then incorporated in to the National Anesthesia Clinical Outcomes Registry, which includes more than 22 million cases from individual practitioners, hospitals, and anesthesia practices (http://www.aqihq.org/airs/airsintro.aspx). This system has gained wide acceptance and participation; as of 2014, 25% of all anesthesia cases in the United States were captured by this system. (5 Years of AQI-What Do We Know About Ourselves Now?) This system collects data on adverse airway events and the total number of anesthesia cases in an ongoing database, allowing for the calculation of the incidence of airway events, and these rates can be followed over time. In 2014 the Anesthesia Quality Institute and the Society of Airway Management established a formalized relationship through a letter of understanding. This provides for an analysis of this substantial database by airway specialists. However, this database is not of use for maintaining individual patient data.

Database Factors: Access, Limited; Timeframe, Ongoing; Denominator, Included.

Type III: Combined Patient Protective, Epidemiologic, and Etiologic Difficult Airway Database

These databases are organized to identify and protect individual patients while also cataloging difficult airway events for epidemiologic and etiologic analysis. This requires recording and storing patient identifiers associated with the airway event information and management data. Additionally, this type of system facilitates data access by future airway providers and should ideally provide patients with airway information.

MedicAlert Foundation: difficult airway/intubation registry

Founded in 1956, the MedicAlert Foundation is a 501(c)3 nonprofit organization that innovated a national and international emergency medical identification emblem and

24/7 emergency response system. MedicAlert Foundation was endorsed by the ASA in 1979, the World Federation of Societies of Anaesthesiologist in 1992, and the American Academy of Otolaryngology-Head and Neck Surgeons in 1993.

In 1992, an Anesthesia Advisory Council comprised of anesthesiologists, otolaryngologists, and experts in safety and risk management joined with the nonprofit MedicAlert Foundation to establish the MedicAlert National Registry for Difficult Airway/Intubation (Andrew Wigglesworth, personal communication, 2010). The major objectives of the MedicAlert Anesthesia Advisory Council were to (1) develop mechanisms for uniform documentation and dissemination of critical airway information, (2) establish a database to store and transmit protected patient information between the MedicAlert Foundation and health care facilities (nationally and internationally), and (3) determine through clinical practice if dissemination of clinical airway information could prevent future adverse outcomes and lower health care costs. A specialty enrollment form for the MedicAlert National Registry for Difficult Airway/Intubation was designed that included a "Dear Patient" panel, "Dear Practitioner" panel, airway database, legal statement, and information for patient enrollment.

In 1994, the Anesthesia Advisory Council reported 111 patient enrollments into the Registry and highlighted potential benefits of enrollment and patient information exchange: anticipation of a difficult airway resulted in fewer techniques used and a lower incidence of adverse outcomes (L.J. Mark and coworkers, unpublished data, 1994). In 1995, in conjunction with the foundation of the Society for Airway Management (SAM), the Anesthesia Advisory Council established a Special MedicAlert Task Force within SAM to oversee the Registry.

Between 1992 and 2014, there were nearly 12,000 patient enrollments in the Registry. In a preliminary survey of these patient enrollments, more than 150 health care institutions from all 50 states are represented. Institutions include freestanding clinics, community hospitals, tertiary care centers, teaching institutions, and military institutions. Approximately 12% of these enrollments included "Dear Patient" letters from their health care providers. Review of these letters identified three broad categories of patient information: (1) generic "difficult airway/intubation alert" only, (2) generic "difficult airway/intubation alert" supplemented with database elements further describing the nature of the difficult airway, and (3) either category one or two with scanned original documentation from the patient's medical record (eg, anesthesia operating room records, surgical operative notes).

In response to this comprehensive review, in 2014, the SAM MedicAlert Task Force updated the National Difficult Airway/Intubation brochure and registry form (http://www.medicalert.org/everybody/difficult-airwayintubation-registry). Health care providers from any background or location can document specified patient airway factors, management techniques, and airway outcomes via a World Wide Web–based system. The providers can either download the registry form and complete it and give it to the patient along with a "Dear Patient" letter (see example), or assist patients with on-line registration. This information is securely stored for patients to access and patients can avail themselves of official MedicAlert medical identification notifying health care providers of their airway status. This information can then be used to provide the appropriate airway management for that patient, without having to locate and contact the prior health care provider.

Both the SAM and the Canadian Airway Focus Group recommend the use of a national registry, such as MedicAlert, in addition to their documentation of a patient's difficult airway.[11,12]

Database Factors: Access, Global; Timeframe, Ongoing; Denominator, None.

CLINICAL PRACTICES AND PATIENT IDENTIFICATION

The 2003 ASA Practice Guidelines for Management of the Difficult Airway contained a difficult airway algorithm that described in great detail the choices and techniques available and the pathways for the management of the unanticipated or anticipated difficult airway/intubation.[13] Subsequent ASA editorials suggested that successful airway techniques and devices would vary, depending on the clinical setting, the skill and experience of the practitioner, and unique characteristics of the patient.[14] How then can these many variations, successful and unsuccessful, be communicated to the next health care provider?

It is also known that repeated attempts at intubation cause swelling and bleeding, with each attempt increasing the likelihood of failed intubation and the possibility of brain damage or even death.[15–17] Prolonged and multiple attempts at intubation can increase the rate of complications up to 70%.[18,19] Given the serious patient safety and liability implications of repeated attempts at intubating the difficult airway patient, how can repeated attempts at intubation be avoided during future events?

The answer to these questions lies in implementing a well-defined, uniform, reliable, and nationally accessible mechanism to document and disseminate critical information about a patient's difficult airway/intubation. The communication of successful and unsuccessful airway management techniques consists of two parts: documentation in the electronic medical record at the time of the event for concurrent providers during that episode of care; and dissemination of that information to the patient and future care providers during subsequent episodes of care.[1]

The ASA Practice Guidelines recommend that "the anesthesiologist should document the presence and nature of the airway difficulty" at the time of the event. This should include "a description of the airway difficulties that were encountered. The description should distinguish between difficulties encountered in face mask or laryngeal mask airway ventilation and difficulties encountered in tracheal intubation." It should also include "a description of the various airway management techniques that were employed. The description itself should indicate the extent to which each of these techniques served a beneficial or detrimental role in management of the difficult airway."[13] The ASA endorses preanesthesia, anesthesia, and postanesthesia documentation, ideally within a special airway management section of the electronic medical record. This section would contain required fields and a comment section for free text.

Many practitioners have put great thought into airway documentation. Combining elements from all of these systems leads to the following list of what to document:

1. Date and institution where difficult airway was identified
2. Provider contact information
3. Patient characteristics on airway examination, body mass index, and other significant comorbidities
4. Type of difficulty encountered with each technique, such as mask ventilation, supraglottic devices, intubation, and extubation
5. Unsuccessful techniques
6. Successful techniques with best view
7. Implications for future
8. Recommendation for registration with Medic Alert[20] (http://www.medicalert.org/difficult-airwayintubation-registry)

Documentation in the Anesthesia Record

Difficult airway documentation should be evident to all care providers. The previous list encompasses the most complete system of difficult airway documentation. Traditionally this was a cover sheet of the patient's paper chart. With the advent of the electronic patient record and the electronic anesthesia record many systems are now being used. One shortcoming of current systems is the inability to transfer difficult airway data automatically from the electronic anesthesia record to the main electronic patient record. Additionally, many electronic systems require that the provider know where to look for difficult airway data, thus hindering all health care providers from obtaining this information (Lynette Mark, MD, personal communication, 2005). Many systems, including that used by the VA, provide the ability to "flag" a patient's chart for a few select conditions. When activated the difficult airway flag appears each time the patient's electronic record is accessed and must be acknowledged before progressing through the rest on the electronic record. This is perhaps the most accurate mimic of the physical face sheet found in paper charts. VA electronic record flags have the added benefit of attaching data to the flag in the face sheet and in a location that is only one layer from the main record page (Jessica Feinleib, personal communication, 2013).

Patient consultation

The 2003 ASA practice guidelines and the VHA recommend that the anesthesiologist notify the patient (or family/responsible party) of the patient's difficult airway/intubation (VHA Directive 2012-032).[13]

Effective notification has usually been interpreted to include verbal and written notification, typically a discussion between the anesthesiologist and the patient delineating the nature of their difficult airway. Anesthesiologists do comply with this recommendation and speak with the patient in the postanesthesia care unit. However, this verbal communication to the patient and/or family may be invalidated because of the patient's postoperative pain, anxiety, or sedation and the family's more immediate concerns about the patient's surgery and recovery as communicated by the surgeon.[21] One study found that 50% of patients informed verbally did not recall or were unsure they had a postoperative conversation with their anesthesiologist.[22] The additional burden of unfamiliar medical words further complicates successful verbal communication of a difficult airway or intubation event. Given all of these factors, a patient reentering a facility may not remember this verbal information and may deny having a history of difficult airway during subsequent preoperative evaluations. The limitations of verbal notification should thus be recognized, particularly with respect to the patient having "a role in guiding and facilitating future care" or being able to accurately disseminate critical information to future health care providers.[13] Thus, the component of verbal communication to the patient is best completed when the patient is alert and oriented or just before being discharged home. The addition of written notification at the time of verbal communication completes the classic patient teaching methods that are used for postoperative instructions.

This process has been formalized in some VA hospitals into a "Difficult Airway Consult" package including patient record flag, patient record note, patient notification letter, and verbal communication with the patient or their designee (VHA Directive 2012-032).

Patient and physician letters

The letter in **Box 1** is a sample provided from the SAM MedicAlert Task Force and can be customized to individual practices. The data entry page for MedicAlert can be found at (www.medicalert.org/difficultairway) (**Box 2**).

Box 1
Difficult airway letter to the patient

[Date]

Dear Patient:

During your recent surgery, you underwent general anesthesia (completely asleep for surgery). This required a breathing tube to be placed in your windpipe to make sure oxygen could get to your lungs, heart, brain, and other vital organs. When the breathing tube was inserted, you were found to have a "DIFFICULT AIRWAY." In other words, it was difficult to place a breathing tube in your windpipe.

Now that we know that you have a "DIFFICULT AIRWAY," it is very important that you do the following to help protect yourself.

1. Tell your primary care physician or family doctor that you have a "DIFFICULT AIRWAY."

2. Tell your family and others of your choosing that you have a "DIFFICULT AIRWAY" in case they need to provide this information on your behalf.

3. If you are to have surgery, tell your anesthesiologist that you have a "DIFFICULT AIRWAY." Show your anesthesiologist the attached form that contains all the medical details needed to manage your difficult airway.

4. You are strongly advised to enroll in the MedicAlert Foundation's Registry for Difficult Airway/Intubation. If you are unable to afford the enrollment fee, please let me know and I can write a letter for a waiver of the fee.

I have informed you of your DIFFICULT AIRWAY because it is extremely important that you are aware of the difficulties in placing a breathing tube. Please keep this letter in a safe place for future reference.

Please contact me if you have any questions or desire further information.

Sincerely.

Your [Anesthesiologist/Health Care Provider]

[Name, Facility, Address, Phone Number]

In-hospital bracelet

The use of bracelets to promote patient identification and safety is now standard of care and endorsed by the World Health Organization and the International Joint Commission (http://www.who.int/patientsafety/solutions/patientsafety/PS-Solution2.pdf). The extension of this highly successful patient safety initiative to denote critical patient comorbidities with color-coded bands is often used. However, there is only marginal standardization as to what the colors indicate (http://endurid.com/blog/2013/06/the-5-different-colors-of-medical-alert-bracelets/). This leads to confusion when staff or patients move between health care systems with different color codes.

The use of an identification bracelet for difficult airway could increase patient safety, but is more effective if they state the patient's condition in text form. This is often seen as a potential HIPAA violation and therefore often not incorporated into a difficult airway patient bracelet system. The use of MedicAlert bracelets to inform health care providers of patient comorbidities has a long history and is well accepted by patients.

The use of in-hospital difficult airway bracelets can safeguard patients, but must be implemented at the hospital level while being aware of the potential pitfalls. An in-hospital difficult airway bracelet system would never be effective as the only part of a notification system, but only as an additional measure combined with the other elements we have discussed.

Difficult airway registry

Please refer to **Fig. 1** and the section on Difficult Airway Databases for a discussion of this topic.

Box 2
MedicAlert foundation registry for difficult airway/intubation

MedicAlert FOUNDATION   DIFFICULT AIRWAY / INTUBATION REGISTRY
Please complete this form and give to your patient.

Download this form at www.medicalert.org/difficultairway

1. PATIENT INFORMATION

FIRST NAME   LAST NAME

MAILING ADDRESS   CITY   STATE   ZIP

PHONE ☐ Home ☐ Mobile ☐ Work   ☐ Home ☐ Mobile ☐ Work

EMAIL ADDRESS

☐ Male ☐ Female

DATE OF BIRTH (MM/DD/YYYY)   GENDER

2. PHYSICIAN & HOSPITAL INFORMATION

FIRST NAME   LAST NAME

PROFESSIONAL TITLE AND SPECIALITY

HOSPITAL/FACILITY   PHONE

ADDRESS   CITY   STATE   ZIP

PATIENT'S MEDICAL RECORD NUMBER

3. DIFFICULT AIRWAY/INTUBATION EVENT DETAILS

WHAT WAS THE OPERATIVE PROCEDURE AND DATE?

PROCEDURE   MO/DAY/YR

WAS THE OPERATIVE PROCEDURE ELECTIVE OR NON-ELECTIVE?
☐ Elective ☐ Non-elective

WHERE DID THE DIFFICULT AIRWAY/INTUBATION EVENT OCCUR?
☐ Hospital operating room
☐ Post-anesthesia care unit/recovery room
☐ Intensive care unit
☐ Emergency department
☐ Nursing unit or ward
☐ Remote hospital procedure site
☐ Ambulatory surgery center
☐ Other _____

PATIENT HEIGHT AND WEIGHT

HEIGHT (IN. OR CM.)   WEIGHT (LB. OR KG.)

ASA PHYSICAL STATUS
☐ ASA physical status I (normal healthy patient)
☐ ASA physical status II (patient with mild systemic disease)
☐ ASA physical status III (patient with severe systemic disease)
☐ ASA physical status IV (patient with severe systemic disease that is constant threat to life)
☐ ASA physical status V (moribund patient who is not expected to survive without the operation)
☐ ASA physical status E (emergency procedure)

WHAT TYPE OF MONITORING WAS USED?
☐ Capnography
   ☐ Color-change/colorimetric
   ☐ Digital
   ☐ Waveform
☐ Oximetry
☐ None

WAS DIFFICULT AIRWAY/INTUBATION ANTICIPATED?
☐ Yes ☐ No

IF ANTICIPATED, HOW?
☐ airway history given by patient
☐ airway history given by family
☐ prior anesthesia record
☐ prior ENT surgery
☐ prior head and neck radiation
☐ prior airway pathology
☐ documentation in patient's medical record
☐ diagnostic tests
☐ consultations
☐ current physical examination
☐ radiation changes
☐ other _____

WHAT TYPE OF DIFFICULTY WAS ENCOUNTERED? SELECT ALL THAT APPLY.
☐ Mask/ventilation
☐ Supraglattic Airway (SGA)
☐ Intubation
☐ Extubation
☐ Other _____

form continues on next page >

WHAT PATIENT CHARACTERISTICS WERE RELATED TO THE DIFFICULT AIRWAY/ INTUBATION? SELECT ALL THAT APPLY.

- ☐ small mouth opening
- ☐ temporomandibular joint
- ☐ prognathism
- ☐ limited mandibular protrusion
- ☐ beard
- ☐ large tongue
- ☐ dentition/large teeth
- ☐ edentulous
- ☐ redundant or edematous tissue
- ☐ hypertrophied lingual tonsils
- ☐ anterior/superior larynx
- ☐ limited neck extension
- ☐ plastic surg implant in face/neck
- ☐ neck circumference
- ☐ short thyromental distance
- ☐ C-spine instability
- ☐ distorted ENT anatomy
- ☐ Obesity
- ☐ Obstructive sleep apnea
- ☐ Infection
- ☐ Pediatric syndrome
- ☐ Pregnancy
- ☐ Other_____

MOUTH OPENING
- ☐ 1 fingerbreadth
- ☐ 2 fingerbreadths
- ☐ 3 fingerbreadths

THYROMENTAL DISTANCE
- ☐ 1 fingerbreadth
- ☐ 2 fingerbreadths
- ☐ 3 fingerbreadths

NECK EXTENSION
- ☐ Full
- ☐ Limited, >35 degrees
- ☐ Limited, <35 degrees

MODIFIED MALLAMPATI CLASS

- ☐ Modified Mallampati Class I (soft palate, uvula, fauces, pillars, visible)

- ☐ Modified Mallampati Class II (soft palate, uvula, fauces visible)

- ☐ Modified Mallampati Class III (soft palate, base of uvula visible)

- ☐ Modified Mallampati Class IV (only hard palate visible)

KHETERPAL MASK VENTILATION GRADE (IF ATTEMPTED)

- ☐ Kheterpal mask ventilation grade 1 (ventilated by mask)
  - ☐ Spontaneous
- ☐ Kheterpal mask ventilation grade 2 (ventilated by mask with oral airway/ adjuvant with or without muscle relaxant)
  - ☐ Muscle relaxant
- ☐ Kheterpal mask ventilation grade 3 (difficult ventilation [inadequate, unstable, or requiring 2 providers] with or without muscle relaxant)
  - ☐ Muscle relaxant
- ☐ Kheterpal mask ventilation grade 4 (unable to mask ventilate with or without muscle relaxant)
  - ☐ Muscle relaxant

MODIFIED CORMACK-LEHANE GRADE

- ☐ Grade 1 – most of glottic opening is visible
- ☐ Grade 2 - only posterior portion of the glottis or only arytenoid cartilages are visible
- ☐ Grade 3 – only the epiglottis is visible
- ☐ Grade 4 – neither glottis nor epiglottis is visible

---

4. SUCCESSFUL EQUIPMENT TECHNIQUES

WHAT EQUIPMENT/TECHNIQUES WERE SUCCESSFUL IN THE PATIENT'S AIRWAY MANAGEMENT? SELECT ALL THAT APPLY.

- ☐ Awake
- ☐ Asleep
- ☐ Face mask ventilation
- ☐ Oral airway
- ☐ Nasal airway
- ☐ Supraglottic airway (SGA)/extraglottic device (EGD)
  - ☐ Intubating supraglottic airway

- ☐ Direct laryngoscope
  - ☐ Macintosh (Size: ☐ 1 ☐ 2 ☐ 3 ☐ 4)
  - ☐ Miller (Size: ☐ 1 ☐ 2 ☐ 3 ☐ 4)
  - ☐ Other _____
- ☐ Video laryngoscope
  - (Size: ☐ 1 ☐ 2 ☐ 3 ☐ 4)
- ☐ Flexible fiberoptic bronchoscope
  - ☐ Oral
  - ☐ Nasal
- ☐ Endotracheal introducer
  - ☐ Aintree exchange catheter
  - ☐ Optical stylet _____

- ☐ Rigid fiberoptic laryngoscope _____
- ☐ Operative laryngoscope/Rigid laryngoscope
  - ☐ Holinger
  - ☐ Dedo
- ☐ Rigid bronchoscope
- ☐ Retrograde intubation set
- ☐ Cricothyrotomy
- ☐ Tracheotomy
- ☐ Percutaneous tracheostomy
- ☐ Other _____

form continues on next page >

5. UNSUCCESSFUL EQUIPMENT TECHNIQUES

WHAT EQUIPMENT/TECHNIQUES WERE UNSUCCESSFUL IN THE PATIENT'S AIRWAY MANAGEMENT? SELECT ALL THAT APPLY.

❑ None

Number of attempts ❑ 1   ❑ 2   ❑ >3

❑ Awake

❑ Asleep

❑ Face mask ventilation

❑ Oral airway

❑ Nasal airway

❑ Supraglottic airway (SGA)/extraglottic device (EGD)

  ❑ Intubating supraglottic airway

❑ Direct laryngoscope

  ❑ Macintosh (Size: ❑ 1   ❑ 2   ❑ 3   ❑ 4)

  ❑ Miller (Size: ❑ 1   ❑ 2   ❑ 3   ❑ 4)

  ❑ Other _____

❑ Video laryngoscope

  (Size: ❑ 1   ❑ 2   ❑ 3   ❑ 4)

❑ Flexible fiberoptic bronchoscope

  ❑ Oral

  ❑ Nasal

❑ Endotracheal introducer

  ❑ Aintree exchange catheter

  ❑ Optical stylet _____

❑ Rigid fiberoptic laryngoscope _____

❑ Operative laryngoscope/Rigid laryngoscope

  ❑ Holinger

  ❑ Dedo

❑ Rigid bronchoscope

❑ Retrograde intubation set

❑ Cricothyrotomy

❑ Tracheotomy

❑ Percutaneous tracheostomy

❑ Other _____

ESTIMATED TIME FOR AIRWAY MANAGEMENT

❑ 0-15 minutes

❑ 15-30 minutes

❑ 30-60 minutes

❑ Longer than 60 minutes

6. PATIENT OUTCOME

WHAT WAS THE PATIENT OUTCOME? SELECT ALL THAT APPLY. FOR RESEARCH PURPOSES ONLY.

❑ Airway secured and procedure completed

❑ Airway secured but procedure cancelled

❑ No adverse outcome

❑ Cancelled procedure

❑ Desaturation

❑ Aspiration

❑ Cardiovascular compromise/arrest

❑ Cricothyrotomy

❑ Tracheotomy

❑ Percutaneous tracheostomy

❑ Dental trauma

❑ Soft tissue or nasal trauma

❑ Esophageal trauma

❑ Laryngeal trauma

❑ Vocal cord trauma

❑ Tracheal trauma

❑ Barotrauma

❑ Hemorrhage

❑ Other _____

7. SIGNIFICANT EVENTS

PLEASE DESCRIBE THE SIGNIFICANT EVENTS

8. FINAL RECOMMENDATION

FINAL COMMENTS/RECOMMENDATIONS FOR COLLEAGUES?

MedicAlert Foundation is endorsed by the Society for Airway Management.

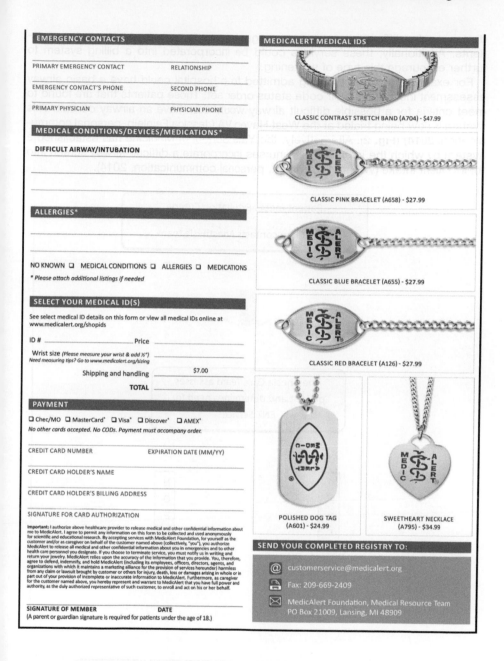

EMERGENCY CONTACTS

PRIMARY EMERGENCY CONTACT   RELATIONSHIP

EMERGENCY CONTACT'S PHONE   SECOND PHONE

PRIMARY PHYSICIAN   PHYSICIAN PHONE

MEDICAL CONDITIONS/DEVICES/MEDICATIONS*

DIFFICULT AIRWAY/INTUBATION

ALLERGIES*

NO KNOWN ☐   MEDICAL CONDITIONS ☐   ALLERGIES ☐   MEDICATIONS
Please attach additional listings if needed

SELECT YOUR MEDICAL ID(S)

See select medical ID details on this form or view all medical IDs online at
www.medicalert.org/shopids

ID # _____ Price _____

Wrist size *(Please measure your wrist & add ½")*
Need measuring tips? Go to www.medicalert.org/sizing

Shipping and handling $7.00

TOTAL _____

PAYMENT

☐ Chec/MO ☐ MasterCard° ☐ Visa° ☐ Discover° ☐ AMEX°
No other cards accepted. No CODs. Payment must accompany order.

CREDIT CARD NUMBER   EXPIRATION DATE (MM/YY)

CREDIT CARD HOLDER'S NAME

CREDIT CARD HOLDER'S BILLING ADDRESS

SIGNATURE FOR CARD AUTHORIZATION

Important: I authorize above healthcare provider to release medical and other confidential information about me to MedicAlert. I agree to permit any information on this form to be collected and used anonymously for scientific and educational research. By accepting services with MedicAlert Foundation, for yourself as the customer and/or as caregiver on behalf of the customer named above (collectively, "you"), you authorize MedicAlert to release all medical and other confidential information about you in emergencies and to other health care personnel you designate. If you choose to terminate service, you must notify us in writing and return your jewelry. MedicAlert relies upon the accuracy of the information that you provide. You, therefore, agree to defend, indemnify, and hold MedicAlert (including its employees, officers, directors, agents, and organizations with which it maintains a marketing alliance for the provision of services hereunder) harmless from any claim or lawsuit brought by customer or others for injury, death, loss or damages arising in whole or in part out of your provision of incomplete or inaccurate information to MedicAlert. Furthermore, as caregiver for the customer named above, you hereby represent and warrant to MedicAlert that you have full power and authority, as the duly authorized representative of such customer, to enroll and act on his or her behalf.

SIGNATURE OF MEMBER   DATE
(A parent or guardian signature is required for patients under the age of 18.)

MEDICALERT MEDICAL IDS

CLASSIC CONTRAST STRETCH BAND (A704) - $47.99

CLASSIC PINK BRACELET (A658) - $27.99

CLASSIC BLUE BRACELET (A655) - $27.99

CLASSIC RED BRACELET (A126) - $27.99

POLISHED DOG TAG
(A601) - $24.99

SWEETHEART NECKLACE
(A795) - $34.99

SEND YOUR COMPLETED REGISTRY TO:

@ customerservice@medicalert.org

Fax: 209-669-2409

MedicAlert Foundation, Medical Resource Team
PO Box 21009, Lansing, MI 48909

Nonoperative patient screening

Most hospitalized patients do not enter the operating room. In this population most patients with difficult airways go undiagnosed. Therefore, efforts should also be made to increase identification of these patients. To this end, nonairway physicians and providers should be educated regarding the negative impact that an unidentified difficult airway can have on a patient's outcomes. All health care providers should be encouraged and educated to assess their patients' airways. They could then obtain airway consultations from airway physicians. These efforts could decrease the discovery of a difficult airway in an emergent scenario and avoid harm to these patients. Additionally, these services could be incorporated into a billing system to further encourage this type of screening.

For example, all patients being admitted to a hospital could have a basic airway assessment included in their code status order set. Those patients that are found to meet criteria for a possible difficult airway would then have an airway consult. This system is now being trialed at the West Haven VA (Jessica Feinleib, personal communication, 2014) (**Fig. 2**). Alternatively, the Yale School of Medicine has established a system by which the intensive care nurses incorporate a difficult airway screen into their patient intake (William Rosenblatt, personal communication, 2014).

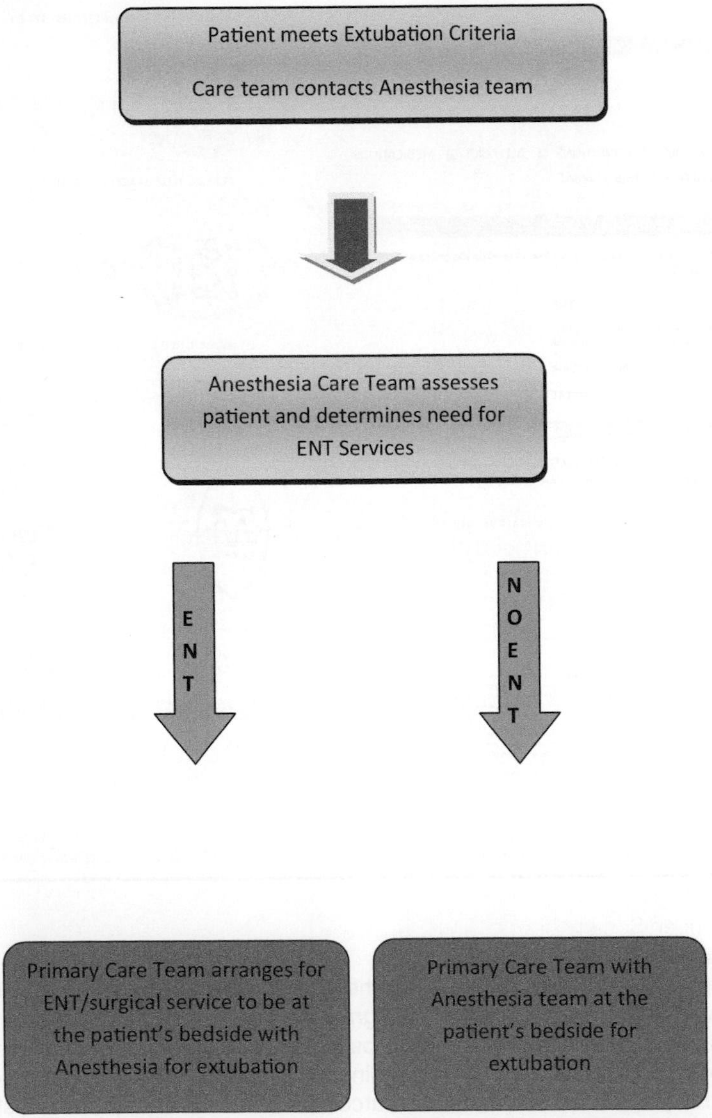

Fig. 2. Algorithm for extubation and intubation of patients with difficult intubation flag. ENT, ear, nose, and throat.

Hospital policies for patients with known difficult airways
After a patient has been diagnosed with a known or likely difficult airway, hospital policies should be in place to support their care in the safest manner. For example, a multidisciplinary group should establish hospital policies regarding the out-of-operating room postoperative estuation, elective intubation, and emergent intubation of these patients. Additionally, procedural sedation of difficult airway patients can place them in jeopardy. These scenarios should be anticipated and systems put in place to safeguard patients.

In summary, the need for a universal, ongoing, fully accessible, and comprehensive patient protective difficult airway database is obvious to all active airway practitioners. In this age of the Internet and "big data," lack of critical information should no longer plague patients and health care practitioners. The ideal database would satisfy all of these requirements while also allowing for the statistical analysis of epidemiologic and etiologic factors that produce unrecognized difficult airways.

FUTURE DIRECTIONS

Although recommendations for difficult airway documentation and data dissemination have existed since the early 1990s, several surveys and studies have shown that such recommendations have not been widely implemented.[20,23,24] One study found that only 20% of anesthesiologists consistently wrote a difficult airway letter to the patient's general practitioner. Of those practitioners that received a difficult airway letter, 98% thought airway information was important but only half forwarded the information to other care providers.[25] A difficult airway letter follow-up survey found that only 50% of patients remembered having a conversation with an anesthesiologist postoperatively, 80% remember getting a letter, 41% of primary providers were aware of the condition, and 23% registered with Medic Alert.[22]

In-hospital difficult airway registries have been shown to decrease emergency surgical airways and empower providers without advanced airway skills to call for assistance earlier in an event.[26,27] Cook and MacDougall-Davis[28] state that "human factors" including communication, judgment, and training, are common factors resulting in airway complications.

In addition to effective difficult airway documentation and communication of this critical information to all relevant health care providers, other measures can further safeguard patient security. These measures include broadening airway screening systems and implementing care policies for patient with documented difficult airways. These are evolving areas and as such little research has been done evaluating their effectiveness in supporting patient care.

REFERENCES

1. Hagberg CA. Benumof and Hagberg's airway management. 3rd edition. Philadelphia: Elsevier; 2012 [chapter: 54].
2. American Society of Anesthesiologists Task Force on Guidelines for Management of the Difficult Airway. Practice Guidelines for management of the difficult airway. Anesthesiology 1993;78:597–602.
3. Caplan RA, Posner K, Ward RJ, et al. Adverse respiratory events in anesthesia: a closed claims analysis. Anesthesiology 1990;72:828.
4. Wilson ME, Spiegelhalter D, Robertson JA, et al. Predicting difficult intubation. Br J Anaesth 1988;61:211.
5. Rose DK, Cohen MM. The airway problem and predictors in 18,500 patients. Can J Anaesth 1989;41:372.

6. Cooper JB, Newbower RS, Long CD, et al. Preventable anesthesia mishaps: a study of human factors. Anesthesiology 1978;49(6):399–406.
7. El-Ganzouri A, McCarthy R, Tuman KJ, et al. Preoperative airway assessment: predictive value of a multivariate risk index. Anesth Analg 1996;82:1197–204.
8. Lundstrom L, Moller A, Rosenstock C, et al. A documented previous difficult tracheal intubation as a prognostic test for a subsequent difficult tracheal intubation in adults. Anaesthesia 2009;64:1081–8.
9. Metzner J, Posner KL, Lam MS, et al. Closed claims' analysis. Best Pract Res Clin Anaesthesiol 2011;25(2):263–76.
10. Pearce A, Shaw J. Airway assessment and planning. In: Cook T, editor. NAP4 Major complications of airway management in the United Kingdom. London: The Royal College of Anaesthestists and the Difficult Airway Society; 2011. p. 135–42.
11. Crosby ET, Cooper RM, Douglas MJ, et al. The unanticipated difficult airway with recommendations for management. Can J Anaesth 1998;45:757–76.
12. Law JA, Broemling N, Cooper RM, et al. The difficult airway with recommendations for management. Part 1: difficult tracheal intubation encountered in an unconscious/induce patient. Can J Anaesth 2013;60:1089–118.
13. American Society of Anesthesiologists Task Force on Management of the Difficult Airway Updated Report. Practice guidelines for management of the difficult airway. Anesthesiology 2003;98:1260–77.
14. American Society of Anesthesiologists Task Force on Management of the Difficult Airway Updated Report. Practice guidelines for management of the difficult airway. Anesthesiology 2013;118:251–70.
15. Orebaugh SL. Difficult airway management in the emergency department. J Emerg Med 2002;22:31–48.
16. Benumof JL. Difficult laryngoscopy: obtaining the best view. Can J Anaesth 1994; 41:361–5.
17. Peterson GN, Domino KB, Caplan RA, et al. Management of the difficult airway: a closed claims analysis. Anesthesiology 2005;103:33–9.
18. Mort T. Emergency tracheal intubation: complications associated with repeated laryngoscopic attempts. Anesth Analg 2004;99:607–13.
19. Combes X, Jabre P, Margenet A, et al. Unanticipated difficult airway management in the prehospital emergency setting. Anesthesiology 2011;114: 105–10.
20. Barron FA, Ball DR, Jefferson P, et al. "Airway alerts." How UK anaesthetists organize, document and communicate difficult airway management. Anaesthesia 2003;58:50–83.
21. Koenig HM. No more difficult airway, again! Time for consistent standardized written patient notification of a difficult airway. APSF Newsletter 2010;p1–6.
22. Trentman TL, Frasco PE, Milde LN. Utility of letters sent to patients after difficult airway management. J Clin Anesth 2004;16:247–61.
23. Mellado P, Thunedborg L. Anaesthesiological airway management in Denmark: assessment, equipment and documentation. Acta Anaesthesiol Scand 2004;48: 350–4.
24. Baker P, Moore L, Hopley L, et al. Dissemination of critical airway information. Anaesth Intensive Care 2013;42:334–41.
25. Wilkes M, Beattie C. Difficult airway communication between anesthesia and the general practitioner. Scott Med J 2013;58:2–6.
26. Sheeran P, Walsh B, Finley AM, et al. Management of difficult airway patients and the use of a difficult airway registry at a tertiary care pediatric hospital. Paediatr Anaesth 2014;24:819–24.

27. Berkow L, Greenberg R, Kan KH, et al. Need for emergency surgical airway reduced by a comprehensive difficult airway program. Anesth Analg 2009;109: 1860–9.
28. Cook T, MacDougall-Davis S. Complications and failure of airway management. Br J Anaesth 2012;109:i68–85.

Index

Note: Page numbers of article titles are in **boldface** type.

Anesthesiology Clin 33 (2015) 415–426
http://dx.doi.org/10.1016/S1932-2275(15)00040-3
1932-2275/15/$ – see front matter © 2015 Elsevier Inc. All rights reserved.
anesthesiology.theclinics.com

Moving?

Make sure your subscription moves with you!

To notify us of your new address, find your **Clinics Account Number** (located on your mailing label above your name), and contact customer service at:

Email: journalscustomerservice-usa@elsevier.com

800-654-2452 (subscribers in the U.S. & Canada)
314-447-8871 (subscribers outside of the U.S. & Canada)

Fax number: 314-447-8029

Elsevier Health Sciences Division
Subscription Customer Service
3251 Riverport Lane
Maryland Heights, MO 63043

*To ensure uninterrupted delivery of your subscription, please notify us at least 4 weeks in advance of move.

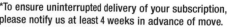

Moving?

Make sure your subscription moves with you!

To notify us of your new address, find your Clinics Account **Number** (located on your mailing label above your name) and contact customer service at:

Email: journalscustomerservice-usa@elsevier.com

800-654-2452 (subscribers in the U.S. & Canada)
314-447-8871 (subscribers outside of the U.S. & Canada)

Fax number: 314-447-8029

Elsevier Health Sciences Division
Subscription Customer Service
3251 Riverport Lane
Maryland Heights, MO 63043

Printed and bound by CPI Group (UK) Ltd, Croydon, CR0 4YY

21/10/2024

01776725-0001